Louis Pasteur's Library: An Unresolved Mystery

Louis Pasteur's Library: An Unresolved Mystery

Armond S. Goldman, MD, Sarita B. Oertling,

Robert O. Marlin IV, MSIS, Kelly L. Caldwell, MLIS

EHDP Press 2019

Louis Pasteur's Library: An Unresolved Mystery

Armond S. Goldman, MD, Sarita B. Oertling, Robert O. Marlin IV, MSIS, Kelly L. Caldwell, MLIS

Cover Image: *Pasteur: The Chemist Who Transformed Medicine*, "The History of Medicine" by Robert Thom circa 1952. Collection of the University of Michigan Health System, Gift of Pfizer, Inc. It depicts the flasks Pasteur used to disprove the spontaneous generation of life and it shows the portraits that Pasteur painted of his parents. Also pictured is Pasteur's wife, Madame Marie Pasteur.

ISBN-13: 978-1-939824-04-2

EHDP Press

Table of Contents

Figures

Dedication

We dedicate this book to members of our families who encouraged us to begin and complete this task.

Acknowledgements

We are grateful for the information generously provided by the following individuals. They were: 1) Daniel Lewis, PhD, the Dibner Senior Curator, History of Science and Technology and Head of the Manuscripts Department at The Huntington Library, Art Collections and Botanical Gardens San Mateo, California; 2) Margaret Tenney, Head of the Reading Room of The Harry Ransom Center of the University of Texas in Austin, Texas; 3) Philip Weimerskirsch, former Associate Director of the Burndy Library; 4) Jeremy Norman, the owner of Jeremy Norman's HistoryofScience.com in Novato, California; 5) Michael Flannery, Curator, and 6) Margaret Balch of the Reynolds Historical Library at the University of Alabama at Birmingham; 7) Sabine Arnaud, PhD, *Forschungsgruppe-Direktor das Max Planck Institute für die Geschichte der Wissenschaft in Berlin*, Deutschland; 8) Sandra Legout, *Médaithèque scientifique de l'Institut Pasteur*; 9) Stéphanie Colin and 10) Muriel Hilaire (*Curateur*) *de Pasteur l'Musée Pasteur a l'Institut Pasteur*; 11) Marie-Laure Prévost and 12) Jérôme Petit *du Département Sciences et techniques du Bibliothèque nationale de France*; 13) Lilla Vekerdy, Head of Special Collections, Smithsonian Libraries, The Dibner Library of the History of Science and Technology; 14) Brent Dibner, President, Dibner Maritime Associates, Chester Hill, Massachusetts and Chairman of the Dibner Institute for the History of Science and Technology at the Massachusetts Institute of Technology, Cambridge, Massachusetts; and the 15) Moody Foundation of Galveston, Texas.

We also thank Professor Heather Green Wooten, PhD, Adjunct Assistant Professor in the Institute of Medical Humanities at the University of Texas Medcial Branch at Galveston for her helpful review of the manuscript.

We appreciate the support that we received from the University of Texas Medical Branch at Galveston and the Moody Medical Library at that medical school.

Finally, this book could not have been completed without the expert editorial assistance of Daniel A. Goldman, MD, MPH.

Most Important Persons in This Story

Louis Pasteur and His Family

Jean Joseph Pasteur and Jeanne Etiennette Roqui - His parents

Marie Pasteur - His wife (née Laurent)

Marie Louise Pasteur - His only surviving daughter

René Vallery-Radot - His son-in-law and biographer

Joseph Louis Pasteur Vallery-Radot - His only grandchild and keeper of his Library

His Educators in Science

Jean-Baptiste Biot - Physics

Antoine Jérôme Balard - Chemistry

Auguste Laurent - Crystallography

His Colleagues in Research

Charles Chamberlain - Chicken cholera, anthrax, and rabies vaccines

Émile Roux - Anthrax and rabies vaccines

Jacque-Joseph Grancher - Rabies vaccine

Book Dealers

Schuman Rare Books in New York City

David Feldman, the House of El Dieff in New York City

Alain Brieux Rare Books in Paris, France

François Chamonal in Paris, France

Jeremy Norman Rare Books and Manuscripts in San Francisco, California

Bibliophiles

Lawrence Reynolds - Radiologist

Harry Huntt Ransom - Humanist

Bern Dibner - Electrical Engineer

Haskell Norman - Psychiatrist

Truman Blocker - Plastic Surgeon

Timeline of the Major Milestones in Pasteur's Career

1847 Graduates from *l'Ecole Normale Supérieur en Paris* with *Docteur-ès-Sciences.*

1849 *Professeur de Chimie ã Strasbourg* in Alsace, France. Demonstrates the chiral properties of certain organic molecules.

1854 *Professeur et Doyen de la Faculté de la Science ã Lille.*

1855 *Professeur de Chimie ã l'Sorbonne* and *Directeur du Laboratoire de la Physico-chimie.*

1862 Disproves the notion of spontaneous generation of life.

1866 Discovers that fermentation that spoils wine is due to microorganisms that in turn are destroyed by controlled heating. Discovers anaerobiosis.

1870 Finds that silkworm disease is due to two separate kinds of infectious agents.

1880 Develops the first laboratory-derived vaccine against chicken cholera.

1881 Develops a vaccine against anthrax infections in sheep.

1886 Develops the first vaccine against a human pathogen: the rabies virus.

1887 Establishes the famed scientific institution that still bears his name, *l' Institut Pasteur.*

Timeline of the Journey of *la Bibliothèque de Louis Pasteur*

1950s   Lawrence Reynolds acquires Louis Pasteur's correspondence with Louis Thuillier possibly from Schuman Rare Books, Ltd. in New York City.

1955   Reynolds donates letters to University of Alabama School of Medicine.

1960s   Parisian rare book dealer, Alain Brieux acquires part of *la Bibliothèque* from Louis Pasteur Vallery-Radot.

1964   Louis Pasteur Vallery-Radot donates most of his grandfather's collection including his laboratory notebooks to *La Bibliothèque Nationale en France*.

~1967   Harry Ransom purchases part of *la Bibliothèque de Louis Pasteur* from Lew David Feldman, the House of El Dieff, in New York City.

1970s   Bern Dibner acquires part of *la Bibliothèque* from Alain Brieux.

~1970   François Chamonal acquires part of *la Bibliothèque* from Vallery-Radot.

~1970   Haskell F. Norman acquires part of *la Bibliothèque* from Chamonal.

1971   J. Norman given his father's part of *la Bibliothèque*.

1977   Moody Foundation acquires Norman's part of *la Bibliothèque* for the University of Texas Medical Branch at Galveston (UTMB).

2006   Huntington Library in San Mateo acquires Dibner's part of *la Bibliothèque*.

2009   Moody Foundation gives their part of *la Bibliothèque* to UTMB.

Chapter 1. Prologue

"It is a great thing to start life with a small number of really good books which are your very own." ~ Sir Arthur Conan Doyle

Before reading this book, if you were asked where the private library of Louis Pasteur (*la Bibliothèque de Louis Pasteur*) is located, you would most likely have responded without too much forethought as we would have done in the early 1970s. Like good Pavlovian primates, we would have confidently stated that his library was safely located in the museum of *l'Institut Pasteur en Paris*, *l'Bibliothèque nationale de France*, or some other national repository in Paris, France. If you came to that seemingly logical conclusion, you would have been wrong. For most of *la Bibliothèque de Louis Pasteur* resides not only outside of Paris, but also outside of France.

The fate of *la Bibliothèque de Louis Pasteur* is a grand, convoluted story that involves famous individuals. In contrast to fictional mysteries, the tale is about real people and how they were responsible for the dispersal of this famous library. Thus, it will be important not only to trace the timing and the route of the dispersal of the library, but also to learn about the lives of the individuals who were involved in this labyrinthine story.

This book concerning the mysterious fate of Pasteur's Library was an outgrowth of our 2014 article on this subject that appeared in the *Journal of Medical Biography*

(1). In that article, many salient features of the fate of Pasteur's library were described. But soon after the article was accepted, new information emerged. Thus, there was far more to the story than could be presented in a journal article. That includes an understanding of the circumstances that led to the library's dispersal, the details of the lives of the major characters in this engaging story, and the fate of *la Bibliothèque de Louis Pasteur* during the Second World War.

In addition, to understand the importance and curious fate of *la Bibliothèque de Louis Pasteur*, it is important first to recall the life, career, and discoveries of its creator, one of the most revered scientists of all time (Figure 1) (Timeline 1). For in some ways the complexity of Pasteur is reflected in the contents of his original library. In turn, the contents of his library may provide some clues to his persona as well as his scientific preoccupations and achievements.

After recounting the life and accomplishments of Pasteur, we will deal with the fate of his library. As you will find, our exploration of the question began four decades ago because of the efforts of a great leader of the institution in which we work. And then many years later, our search greatly expanded when we discovered that other sections of Pasteur's library were in other parts of the United States. Key individuals in those institutions gave freely of their time and knowledge to help us learn how and perhaps why *la Bibliothèque de Louis Pasteur* had been dispersed.

Then we will explore the gifted individuals who obtained the several parts of *la Bibliothèque de Louis Pasteur*. We asked the following questions concerning them.

What was the uniqueness of each of them? What did they have in common? What did they know about Pasteur? What led each of them to appreciate medical history and to obtain an important part of *la Bibliothèque de Louis Pasteur*?

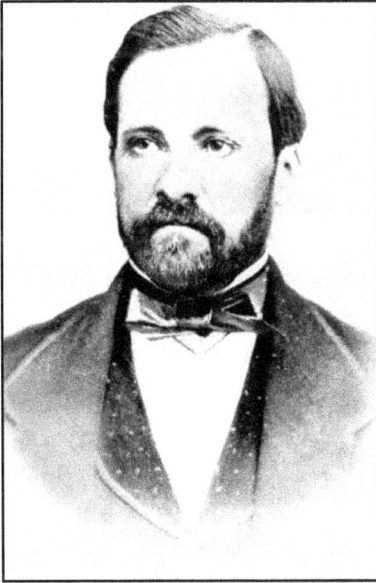

Figure 1a. Louis Pasteur. Age 35
(1857)

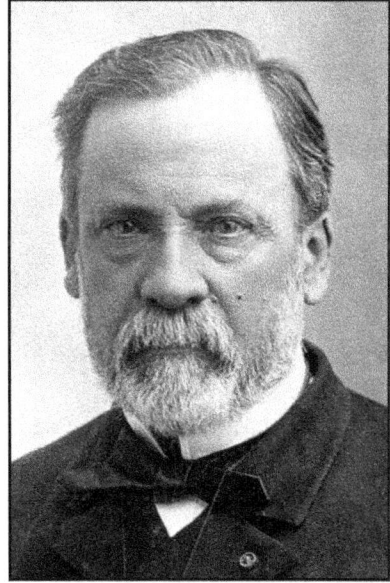

Figure 1b. Louis Pasteur. ~ Age 68
(Circa 1890)

Finally, we will pose the still unanswered questions concerning the intriguing fate of *la Bibliothèque de Louis Pasteur* and indicate why those questions are important. In that respect, it has been a half-century since Pasteur's Library began to be dispersed and nearly all of the participants involved in the dispersal have long since passed away. So now, one has to rely upon secondary sources to complete the task, and some of them could be readers of this book.

Chapter 2. Life and Accomplishments of Louis Pasteur

"It is surmounting difficulties that makes heroes." ~ Louis Pasteur

"The future belongs to Science. More and more she will control the destinies of the nations. Already she has them in her crucible and on her balances."
~ Sir William Osler in *The Life of Pasteur*

To understand the mysteries surrounding *la Bibliothèque de Louis Pasteur*, it is necessary to learn how Pasteur emerged as one of the key innovators, if not the founder of the sciences of microbiology and immunology. This is particularly relevant, since based upon his humble beginnings, his childhood, and the state of biological sciences at the time of his birth, virtually no one would have predicted that would happen. This exploration will begin with a brief exposé of the development of the physical and biological sciences that preceded Pasteur and provided a basis for his research.

Prelude to Pasteur's Life in Science

Long before Pasteur began his illustrious career in science, prestigious universities had been established in several Western European countries including Italy, Germany, England, Sweden, and France. Religion, law, civil affairs, medicine, and science were emphasized. The first such institution in France was *l'Université de Paris* (circa 1160–1250). The emphasis upon science varied considerably depending upon the faculty and facilities in each institution. Be that as it may, the possibilities in Western Europe to become a scientist who might make scientific discoveries, particularly in the physical sciences and mathematics, grew over time. Therefore, by the nineteenth century, there were many more opportunities for students who had the inclinations and the financial resources for an education in a scientific discipline. In parallel, scientists who made the new discoveries often used methods from other aspects of science for their research, modified laboratory equipment for their experiments, or innovated new methods for their endeavors.

The Printing Press

The extensive use of the printing press accelerated the dissemination of scientific knowledge. Although the printing press was developed in China in about 1041, it had little practical impact until about 1450 when the German blacksmith, goldsmith, and publisher, Johannes Gensfleisch zur Laden zum Gutenberg, developed a printing system that mass-produced books and journals in a relatively short period of time (2). To do so, Gutenberg modified the construction of the printing system so that the pressing power exerted by the plate on the paper was evenly applied. To speed up the printing process, Gutenberg also introduced a movable under-table with a plane surface on which the paper sheets could be swiftly changed. His use of an oil-based ink was also an important innovation. This type of printing press quickly spread throughout Europe and provided students more affordable, up-to-date books for their education. Furthermore, it greatly speeded communications between scientists and remained the chief mode of communication until the digital age.

The increased spread of scientific information between countries galvanized the development of science. Subsequently, a critical mass of scientists in certain fields led to the creation of specialized journals that contained the latest findings from researchers in particular fields. So even when a scientist could not travel to a distant country, his or her research findings could be transmitted, not instantaneously as in the present digital age, but nevertheless within a matter of weeks to distant universities and other sites where other researchers worked. Consequently, preexisting libraries expanded, and new ones were created in academic institutions. Moreover, individual scientists or other interested parties began to collect books, journals, and other writings according to their interests. As we discuss later, some of those libraries became phenomenally large and were later given to institutions of higher learning.

Physical Scientists

The development of institutions of higher learning and the provisions for scientists to devote themselves to research in the fields of their interest allowed many remarkable advances in science occurred in Europe long before Pasteur appeared on the scene. Two of the luminaries were Galileo Galilei (1564-1642) and Sir Isaac Newton (1642-1727).

In a certain sense, Galileo founded modern science by his astronomical discoveries that changed the emphasis from a geocentric model (earth was the center of the universe) to a heliocentric model (the sun was the center of the universe) and thus created a more accurate picture of the world. Isaac Newton, who was born in the year that Galileo died, laid the foundations of classical mechanics and formulated the laws of motion and universal gravity. Indeed, those fundamental discoveries were necessary for others to begin to ponder and experiment in physics and mathematics.

Microscopes

It is unclear who invented the microscope. But some were available to explore many aspects of biology by the seventeenth century. The instruments were further developed during the sixteenth and seventeenth centuries and improved upon considerably in the nineteenth century. With them, it became possible for Robert Hooke (1635-1703) from England to visualize that tissues were comprised of cells; for Marcello Malpighi (1628-1694) from Italy to discern complex microscopic structures of a number of organs; and for Antonie Philips van Leeuwenhoek (1632-1723) from the Netherlands to detect spermatozoa, the flow of blood in capillaries, and the presence and multiplication of protozoa and bacteria (animalcules).

Scientists Who Strongly Influenced Louis Pasteur

Other scientific advances during the eighteenth and early nineteenth centuries paved the way for Pasteur to embark upon a career in science. Indeed, he was proverbially the right person at the right place at the right time, and by a stroke of good fortune, funds were provided for his education in an institution of higher learning.

Three pioneer European researchers strongly influenced Pasteur during his formative years in science. They were Joseph Priestley (1733-1804), Antoine-Laurent de Lavoisier (1743-1794), and Pierre-Simon Laplace (1749-1827). Although Priestley had little formal education in science, this famous English clergyman, natural philosopher, chemist, educator, and grammarian discovered several "airs" (gases) (3). Some argued that Priestley was handicapped by not having a formal education in science. But on the other hand, he entered the field of experimentation without the burden of preconceived notions that might have precluded the experiments he performed.

Priestley helped to discover the airs including nitrous air (nitric oxide); vapor of spirit of salt, later called acid air (anhydrous hydrochloric acid); alkaline air (ammonia); diminished or dephlogisticated nitrous air (nitrous oxide); and, most famously, dephlogisticated air (oxygen). These experiments helped to repudiate the last vestiges of the theory of four elements and set the stage for further discoveries of chemical elements and chemical reactions.

The renowned French scientist Antoine-Laurent de Lavoisier worked at the same time when Priestley was discovering several gases. In contrast to Priestley, Lavoisier received an excellent, broad education in the sciences. At the *Collège des Quatre-Nations* (also known as *Collège Mazarin*) in Paris, France, he studied chemistry, botany, astronomy, and mathematics. Lavoisier examined the properties of oxygen and hydrogen, established that sulfur was an element, predicted the existence of silicon as a component of quartz, helped construct the metric system, and organized the first extensive list of elements. Working with Pierre-Simon Laplace, Lavoisier conducted a series of experiments that demonstrated that respiration in mammals provided atmospheric oxygen for a slow combustion of endogenous organic compounds. Although he did not discover other elements, his work clarified the nature of an element.

Lavoisier also performed some of the first quantitative chemical analyses. In those classical experiments, he carefully weighed the chemical reactants in a container and the products that formed in a chemical reaction while in that same container. He showed that although the state of matter changed during the chemical reaction, the total mass of matter did not change. That possibly influenced Pasteur's thinking about the question of spontaneous generation of life.

Lavoisier's *Traité élémentaire de chimie* (Elementary Treatise on Chemistry) (4) is considered to be the first modern chemistry textbook. In that book, he presented a unified view of the new theories of chemistry, a clear statement of the conservation of matter, and a reasoned denial of the existence of phlogiston, a fire-like element that was believed for centuries to be common to combustible materials. In addition, Lavoisier clarified the concept that an element was a substance that could not be broken down by any known chemical process and that chemical compounds formed from combinations of elements. Surely, Pasteur carefully studied that book.

Finally, there was Pierre-Simon Laplace (5), who was perhaps the most phenomenal scientist of his time. Like Pasteur, Laplace rose from humble beginnings. His father,

Pierre, was a farmer and a cider merchant in Beaumont-en-Auge, Normandy, France. Laplace attended a school in the village run by a Benedictine priory. At age sixteen, because of his high intelligence and devotion to the church, Laplace went to the University of Caen in Lower Normandy to read theology and to become a priest in the Roman Catholic Church. It was during that period that he developed great enthusiasm for mathematics. Consequently, he changed from training for the priesthood to a career in science.

Because of his aptitude for mathematics, Laplace was afforded a chance to be interviewed by the well-known French mathematician and polymath Jean-Baptiste le Rond d'Alembert, who coauthored with Denis Diderot the famous *Encyclopédie, ou dictionnaire raisonné des sciences, des arts et des métiers* (*Encyclopaedia, or a systematic dictionary of the sciences, arts, and crafts*). When d'Alembert tested him, he recognized that Laplace, though still a child, had extraordinary mathematical abilities. D'Alembert therefore recommended that Laplace be appointed to a teaching position in the *École Militaire* in Paris. His career in mathematics and the sciences was thus launched.

Besides Laplace's work on oxygen with Lavoisier, this mathematician, physicist, astronomer formulated mathematical methods, the Laplace's equation and the Laplace transform (a widely used integral transform, a particular type of mathematical operator), that appear in many branches of mathematical physics. Moreover, he further developed Bayes' method of statistics that deals with inferences expressed as prior probabilities. One of his quotes, translated into English, exemplified his sense of mathematics.

One sees, from this Essay, that the theory of probabilities is basically just common sense reduced to calculus; it makes one appreciate with exactness that which accurate minds feel with a sort of instinct, often without being able to account for it.

Laplace is particularly well known for his many discoveries in astronomy, his nebular hypothesis of the origin of the solar system, and his predictions of the existence of black holes and gravitational collapse that were proven during the late twentieth century.

Louis Pasteur's Fame

Without the accomplishments of his illustrious predecessors, Pasteur would have been unable to begin the revolutionary experiments that culminated in the birth of the sciences of stereochemistry, microbiology, and immunology and set the stage for the development of a host of immunizations that dramatically reduced the frequencies of many serious infectious diseases. Thus, in some ways he equaled or surpassed the achievements of his predecessors in science.

In addition to his achievements in three separate branches of science, Pasteur created a research institution that nurtured the development of several other microbiologists and immunologists who would continue to carry the revolutions in microbiology and immunology. Indeed, that institute (Figure 2) supported several brilliant scientists who made notable discoveries. 1) Émile Roux and Andre Yersin discovered diphtheria toxin and developed an antiserum to that toxin. 2) Ilya Ilyich Metchnikoff principally elucidated the nature and biological importance of cellular immunity (6). 3) Jules Bordet discovered complement and antibodies. Antibodies were antigen specific, whereas complement was not but was bound to antigen-antibody complexes. Bordet also discovered the cause of whooping cough (pertussis) (7). 4) Paul-Louis Simond demonstrated that the plague pathogen that was discovered by Yersin (8) was transmitted by fleas (9). 5) Albert Calmette and Camille Guerin developed the first vaccine against *Mycobacterium tuberculosis* (10). 6) Alphonse Laveran discovered the malaria parasites (11). 7) Félix d'Herelle discovered bacteriophages (12). 8) André Michael Lwoff discovered proviruses (the latent form of viruses) (13), and Luc Montagnier, Françoise Barré-Sinoussi, and their colleagues discovered the human immunodeficiency viruses (14) that are widespread in many parts of our world. Moreover, eight scientists from *l'Institut Pasteur* were awarded outright the Nobel Prize in Physiology or Medicine and two more shared the Prize in Physiology or Medicine. Furthermore, the first experiments that established by a filtration method that poliovirus were considerably smaller than bacteria or fungi were conducted at the institute in 1906 by Karl Landsteiner, MD from Vienna, Austria and his collaborator Constantin Levaditi, MD, a member of *l'Institut Pasteur* (15). Thus, long after his death, Pasteur's scientific legacy lived on in the institute he created.

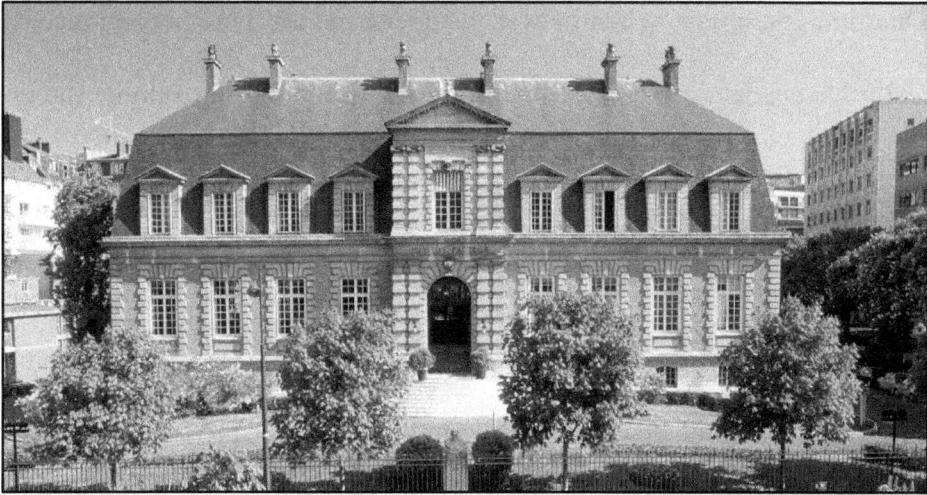

Figure 2. l'Institut Pasteur. The institute created by Louis Pasteur.

Pasteur's founding of three important scientific disciplines - crystallography, infectious diseases, and immunology - established him as one of the most remarkable individuals of his day and inspired not only his immediate colleagues and future scientists at *l'Institut Pasteur en Paris* but also future generations of scientists regardless of the countries of their origin. It was therefore expected that it took a considerable effort to learn not only about Pasteur's remarkable achievements, but also to discover the works in science that he collected; his correspondence with fellow scientists, his friends, and rivals in science; his written comments on the scientific reports written by those friends or rivals; pictures of his colleagues and other notables in his life; and correspondence asking for financial support from the French Government for the institute that he created.

As with many great figures in science, *la Bibliothèque de Louis Pasteur* is a reflection of his thoughts, his scholarship, and his accomplishments. In that respect, Pasteur began building his library when he was a student and the library continued to grow throughout his academic career. It therefore is informative to examine the contents of his library in relation to different periods of his personal and professional life.

Humble Beginnings

Before the *la Bibliothèque de Louis Pasteur* could be conceptually reassembled, it was important to examine how Pasteur rose to fame. It was a proverbial Horatio Alger story, about poor boys, who made good (16). But Pasteur's story exceeded those fantasies in that few who sprang from such humble beginnings achieved such international fame (17, 18). And, the story has certain ironic twists.

Louis Pasteur was born on December 27, 1822 in Dôle, a small village in Eastern France close to the western border of Switzerland. The family name, Pasteur, was probably derived from the French *pâturage*, i.e. pasturage, since they raised and pastured animals for a living. He was descended from a modest family of tanners who lived for most of Pasteur's early years in nearby Arbois, France. His father Jean Joseph Pasteur and his mother Jeanne Etiennette Roqui (Figure 3), a native of Mamoz, France, were married in 1816. He was the third child of his parents. Little is known concerning his family, except that none of them achieved a higher education or became noteworthy.

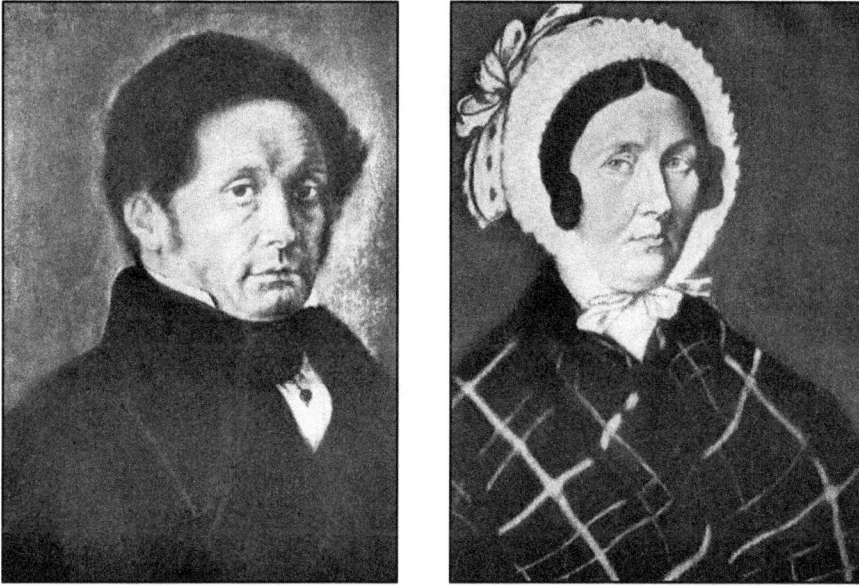

Figure 3. Portraits by Louis Pasteur of His Parents.

Pasteur's parents doted on him, because they sensed that he was unusually intelligent. In turn, Pasteur greatly admired his parents. He was particularly proud that his father Jean Joseph served under Napoleon Bonaparte during the Peninsular War in Spain (military conflict between Napoleon's Empire and Bourbon Spain) from 1812 through 1813. For his bravery, Jean Joseph was awarded France's highest military honor, *Chevalier de la Legion d'honneur (*Knight of the Legion of Honor*)*. The honor given to him imbued in Louis a life-long patriotism that most likely led to his zeal to contribute to French science and perhaps also to doubt the achievements of scientists from certain competing countries.

Although Louis' parents were of modest means and not well educated, they and Monsieur Romanet, the school headmaster of *l'Université d'Arbois* where he received his primary education, recognized that Louis was exceptionally intelligent and was likely capable of attaining great achievements. They therefore encouraged Louis to seek an advanced education in a major university in France. However, that would be difficult because of the expense of such an education. Furthermore, even if the education could be afforded, it was doubtful that he would study science for during childhood he displayed little interest in science or other fields except for portrait painting (16). His artistic talents are exemplified in the existing portraits of his parents (Figure 3) and in his other preserved artwork.

The portraits of Pasteur's parents attest to his keen appreciation of light and perspective. It is curious that there is no indication that he painted scenes from nature, as one might have expected from his future scientific preoccupations. However, there may have been more similarities in science and artistry than differences. Both science and art require imagination, an attention to detail, an ability to synthesize, and great patience. And in both cases, something is created that was not previously obvious. In art, a portrait captured on canvas is the view of the artist. In science, a discovery might be brought to light from experiments designed to test a hypothesis posed by the researcher. In both cases, something is created in the mind before it is visualized. Furthermore, Pasteur's artistic abilities served him in good stead when he was documenting the crystalline nature and chiral properties of certain organic compounds.

Higher Education

Pasteur's parents advised him to seek a profession that was more financially secure than portrait painting. But that would require a higher education in a well-established institution in France, and such an education would be very expensive. Therefore, as much as Pasteur's parents desired the opportunity for their son, they could not afford the great expenses that would entail.

However, aid came from a friend of the family. Captain Barbier in the Parisian municipal guard, who served with Louis' father in the Peninsular War, learned about Louis's need and generously funded his travel, lodgings, and admission to a school in Paris. Therefore, in 1838 Louis moved to the *Institut Barbet* in Paris to begin his higher education.

At first, it seemed that Louis would fail to take advantage of his newly found educational opportunities. He had trouble finding that seemingly intangible something that many in the arts and sciences look for, something that would captivate one's interest. Shortly after he joined the *Institut Barbet*, he became homesick and returned home. After regrouping for some months, he returned to Paris in 1839 and entered the *Collège Royal de Besançon*. One year later, he earned his *Baccalauréat*. He then concentrated on studies in science and obtained a *Baccalauréat Scientifique* (General Science) from Dijon, France.

It was peculiar that Pasteur scored a rather poor grade in chemistry, but that may have been because he found it difficult to adapt to structured academic examinations. His difficulties with some aspects of sciences and with structured examinations were further evident in 1842, when he failed his first attempt to pass the entrance examination for *l'École Normale Supérieure* in Paris. He persisted and succeeded in 1844. In 1845, he received *l'Licencié ès Sciences* (Bachelor of Science) degree.

After Pasteur floundered in his studies, he suddenly awakened to the wonders of physical sciences. This burst of interest appeared to be sparked to a great extent by some of the famous scientists he encountered during his education. They included the famous chemist – crystallographer Auguste Laurent (1808-1853) who discovered anthracene and phthalic acid, characterized carbolic acid, and helped to lay the foundation of organic chemistry (19); the chemist Jean-Baptiste-André Dumas (1800-1884), who studied organic synthesis and atomic weights (20); and the celebrated French physicist, mathematician, astronomer Jean-Baptiste Biot (1774-1862) (21) (Figure 4) who studied the polarization of light, magnetism, astronomy, and the extraterrestrial origin of meteorites.

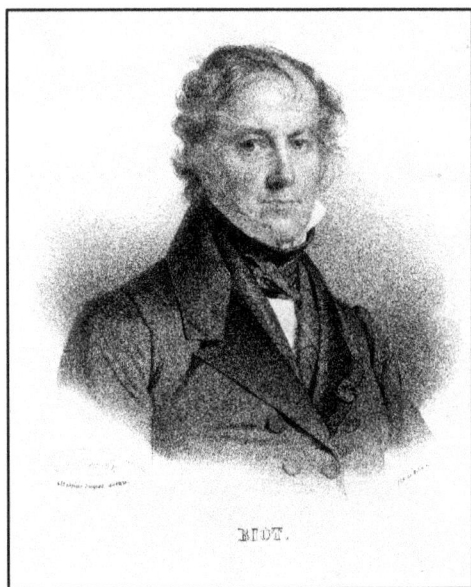

Figure 4. Jean-Baptiste Biot

A famous French physicist, mathematician who inspired Louis Pasteur when Pasteur was in his formative years.

Jean-Baptiste Biot was particularly important in Pasteur's development. He inspired Pasteur and provided the basis for his early studies on the crystalline structures of certain organic crystals. Given that array of luminaries in the physical sciences, it was not surprising that Pasteur decided to become a chemist. There is no evidence that he was interested in biology, and medical sciences were probably even further removed from his mind during those formative years.

Early Research in Crystallography

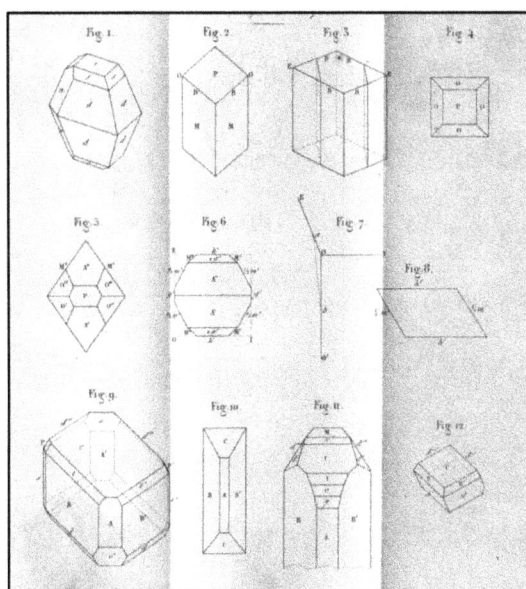

Figure 5. Louis Pasteur's Drawings of Tartaric Acid Crystals

At *l'Ecole Normale*, Pasteur became an assistant to the famous chemist Antoine Jérôme Balard (1802-1876) (22) who discovered bromine in seawater. In Balard's laboratory, Pasteur observed the difference between "right-handed" and "left-handed" crystals of tartaric acid. His discovery concerning crystalline structures of tartaric acid and their chiral nature (non-superimposable mirror images) (Figure 5) became the basis for his later investigations in that field and indirectly led to his subsequent groundbreaking discoveries in microbiology and immunology. Balard also helped Pasteur many years later to devise the fundamental experiments that disproved the spontaneous generation of life.

Start of Louis Pasteur's Academic Career

Pasteur's studies in *l'Ecole Normale Supérieur en Paris* culminated in *Docteur-ès-Sciences* in 1847 at age 25. Because of his early success in crystallography and inspiration of his teachers, Pasteur decided upon an academic career. He quickly attained success in academia. Two years after obtaining his doctorate degree from *l'Ecole Normale Supérieur en Paris*, Pasteur became *Professeur de Chimie ã Strasbourg* in Alsace in Eastern France. Five years later (1854), he moved to *l'Université Lille* in Northern France (French Flanders) where he became the first *Professor et Doyen de la Faculté de la Science ã Lille*. Pasteur's stay there was short for in 1855 he accepted a position in *l'Ecole Normale Supérieur en Paris* where he had previously studied. He also became *Professeur de Chimie ã l'Sorbonne* and *Directeur du Laboratoire de la Physico-chimie*.

During the twenty-two years in those positions, Pasteur made remarkable discoveries that became the basis of the sciences of microbiology and immunology. Then in 1887, he founded the scientific institution that still bears his name, *l'Institut Pasteur en Paris*.

Discovery of Chiral Nature of Certain Organic Compounds

Pasteur's first independent research at the *Université à Strasbourg* concerned the discrepancy between the ability of naturally occurring and synthetic tartaric acid to rotate a beam of light that passed through them. He was fortunate to investigate appropriate molecules, to have the correct temperatures in his laboratory for the experiments concerning the crystalline structures of tartaric acid to succeed, and to have the patience and skill to identify the different populations of crystals by microscopy. Pasteur discovered mirror-image populations of several organic crystals. First, he separated by hand racemic (dextrorotatory and levorotatory forms of a compound in equal proportions) mixtures of tartaric acid crystals into right-handed and left-handed populations. When the tartaric acid crystals were resolubilized, he found that they rotated polarized light to the right or left depending upon their orientation. Thus, Pasteur ascertained by chemistry and physics those optical refractions of the organic molecules - tartaric acid, quinine, and aspartic acid - were not due to different compositions, but to molecular asymmetries (17, 18, 23-26). How these asymmetries developed was unknown, but Pasteur suggested that they were primordial events. By conducting experiments with organic molecules, he was one of the first to forge a link between the physical and biological sciences. Furthermore, his findings spurred investigations by others that demonstrated the chiral nature of many carbon-based, organic compounds.

The Prevailing Theory of Spontaneous Generation of Life

Pasteur conducted a decisive experiment that disproved the ancient notion of the spontaneous generation of all forms of life. The background of this long-standing belief was as follows. Aristotle (Figure 6) fervently believed in the spontaneous generation of life. This is borne out by a quotation from Aristotle's History of Animals, Book V, Part 1 written in about 350 BCE (27).

"Now there is one property that animals are found to have in common with plants. For some plants are generated from the seed of plants, whilst other plants are self-generated through the formation of some elemental principle similar to a seed; and of these latter plants some derive their nutriment from the ground, whilst others grow inside other plants, as is mentioned, by the way, in my treatise on Botany. So with animals, some spring from parent animals according to their kind, whilst others grow spontaneously and not from kindred stock; and of these instances of spontaneous generation some come from putrefying earth or vegetable matter, as is the case with a number of insects, while others are spontaneously generated in the inside of animals out of the secretions of their several organs."

Aristotle added the following in support of the concept of the spontaneous generation in some animals and plants.

"Animals and plants come into being in earth and in liquid because there is water in earth, and air in water, and in all air is vital heat so that in a sense all things are full of soul. Therefore, living things form quickly whenever this air and vital heat are

enclosed in anything. When they are so enclosed, the corporeal liquids being heated, there arises as it were a frothy bubble."

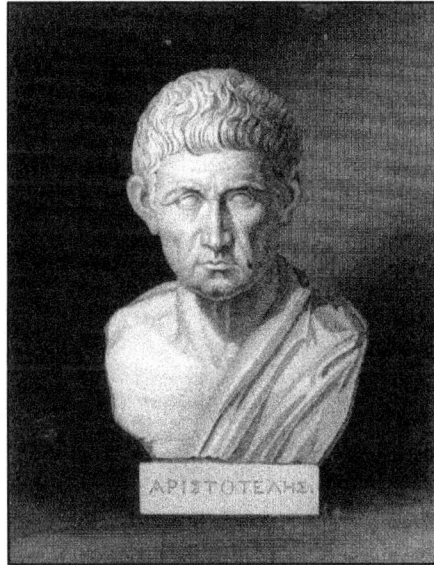

Figure 6. Aristotle. Famous Greek scientist – philosopher.

Aristotle's views were universally believed until the fourteenth century when a few scientists began to doubt it. The English physician William Harvey (1578-1657), who first correctly discerned the human circulatory system, found in his dissections of the uterus of pregnant deer that an embryo was not visible during the first month of pregnancy (28). He correctly surmised that the embryo formed from an invisible ovum. That would not be proven until the early nineteenth century when ova were visualized by microscopic examination (29).

The Flemish scientist Jan Baptist van Helmont's (1580-1644) experimental observations on the growth of plants casted doubt on the belief of spontaneous generation of life (30). Helmont grew a willow tree and measured the amount of soil,

the weight of the tree and the water he added. After five years, the plant gained about

74 kg. Because the amount of soil was basically the same as it had been at the start

of the experiment, he deduced that the tree's weight gain came from water. Since it

had received only water and the soil weighed practically the same as at the beginning,

he concluded that the increased weight of wood, bark and roots formed from water

alone. Helmont's deduction was incomplete, since a large proportion of the mass of

plants comes from atmospheric carbon dioxide that is converted into carbohydrates

via photosynthesis. However, his findings were contrary to the ancient and then

current belief in spontaneous generation of life.

Periodically, certain physicians expressed more enlightened views concerning the

genesis of infectious diseases that was contrary to the belief in spontaneous

generation of life. An important example was the 16th century Veronese physician

and scholar Girolamo Fracastoro (1478-1553) who invented the term syphilis for his

epic poem, *Syphilis sive morbus gallicus* (*Syphilis or "The French Disease"*).

Fracastoro also advanced ideas concerning the nature of infections. He wrote *"I call*

fomites such things as clothes, linen, etc., which although not themselves corrupt, can

nevertheless foster the essential seeds of the contagion and thus cause infection." He

thought, however, that the infectious agents were chemicals rather than living

microorganisms (31).

The belief of spontaneous generation of life was also contrary to the findings of

Francesco Redi (1626-1697), a physician from Tuscany, Italy, who demonstrated in 1668 that maggots did not appear in veal or fish in jars from which adult flies were excluded by a fine mesh gauze (32). His observations included the size of the maggots, but what happened in respect to the much smaller forms of life that we now call microbes was unknown.

It is peculiar that the theory of spontaneous generation of life persisted even after Antonie Philips van Leeuwenhoek (1632-1723) (from the Dutch Republic - the current Netherlands) detected the multiplication of bacteria in 1675. Indeed, the Royal Society in London initially derided van Leeuwenhoek's observations (33), but a few years later his finding were accepted, and he was elected to be a Fellow of the Royal Society.

Thus, despite evidence to the contrary, the belief in spontaneous generation still held sway during the early nineteenth century. One of the chief proponents of spontaneous generation of life during Pasteur's time in the mid nineteenth century was Félix-Archiméde Pouchet (1800-1872), *l'Directeur de l' Museum d'Historie Naturelle de Rouen*. He went so far as to conduct experiments to prove spontaneous generation of microbial agents. He found that microorganisms appeared in boiled hay under mercury exposed to oxygen or air (34). Thus, Pouchet concluded that he had proven that spontaneous generation of life occurred. It was later determined that his experiments were flawed because the mercury was contaminated with spore-forming bacteria (26). Furthermore, at about the same time that Pouchet was conducting his experiments, Charles Cagniard de la Tour, a physicist, and Theodor Schwann, one of the founders of the cell theory, published their independent discoveries of yeast in alcoholic fermentation (35). When they used the microscope to examine foam left over from the process of brewing beer, they observed yeast cells undergoing cell division. Fermentation did not occur when sterile air or pure oxygen was introduced if yeast were absent. This suggested that airborne microorganisms, not spontaneous generation, were responsible for fermentation.

Pasteur Refutes the Theory of Spontaneous Generation of Life

Building upon the 1768 observations by the famous Italian biologist Lazzaro Spallanzani concerning microbes in the air, the demonstration of bacterial multiplication by van Leeuwenhoek, and Charles Cagniard de la Tour and Theodor Schwann's findings concerning fermentation, in the early 1860s Pasteur delivered what many consider to be the final blow to the concept of spontaneous generation of life. In his experiments that were as fundamental as the discovery of the concept of homeostasis by the French physiologist Claude Bernard (1813-1878), swan-necked vessels (Figure 7) were used to exclude dust-borne microorganisms from growth media in flasks. Pasteur may also have been encouraged to do the swan-neck experiments after reading Charles Darwin's 1859 seminal work *On the Origin of Species by Means of Natural Selection or The Preservation of Favoured Races in the Struggle for Life* (36).

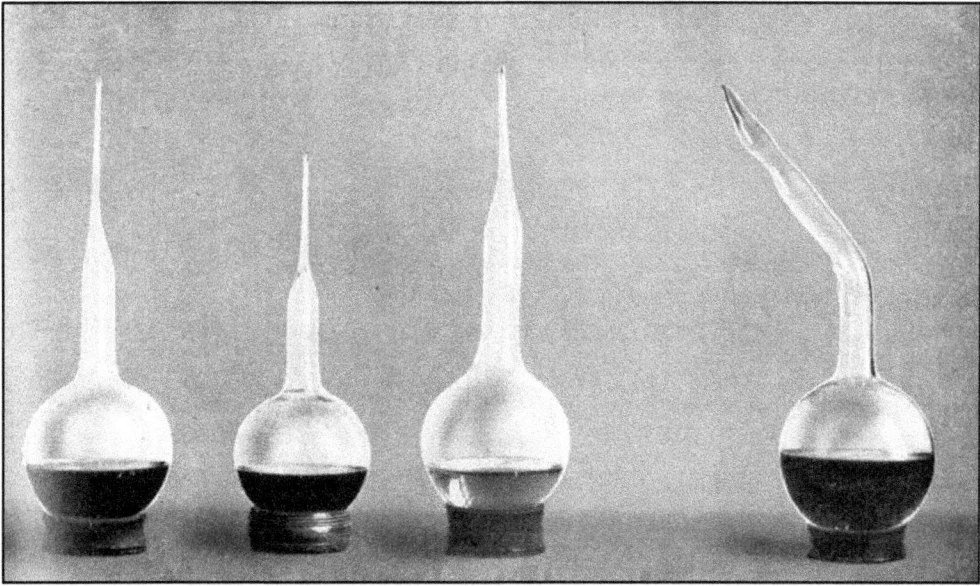

Figure 7. Replicas of Swan-Necked Flasks that Louis Pasteur Used to Disprove Spontaneous Generation of Life.

After preparing a series of glass flasks, he drew out the necks of the vessels into very narrow extensions, curved in various ways and exposed them to the air by an opening one to two millimeters in diameter. Without sealing these flasks, the liquid in some of them was boiled for several minutes. Others that were not boiled served as controls. When all flasks with a straight neck were placed in calm air, the unheated liquids became covered with various molds in twenty-four to forty-eight hours. Moreover, if one of the curved necks was detached from a hitherto sterile flask and placed upright in it, vegetative growths appeared in a few days. Pasteur concluded that the "sinuosities and inclinations" of his swan-necked flasks prevented the liquids from vegetative growths by capturing the dusts that entered with the air. In fact, he insisted, nothing in the air - whether gases, fluids, electricity, magnetism, ozone, or some unknown or occult agent - was a precursor of microbial life except the germs carried by atmospheric dusts (37).

Thus, Pasteur proved that some small infectious agents were airborne, rather than generated spontaneously. These experimental findings strongly suggested that epidemic diseases were caused not by spontaneous creation of microbial life but by microbial agents transmitted by air or by other routes. Thus, the science of microbiology began and the vast world of microbial agents (viruses, bacteria, and protozoans) began to emerge to a group of enlightened scientists led in large part by Pasteur and his colleagues. And that in turn led to exploration of the immune system that protects against microbial pathogens, an exploration that continues to this day.

Early Application of Germ Theory to Prevent Diseases

Fermentation

Pasteur became widely appreciated by other scientists in France because of his scientific successes. Consequently, the French Government asked Pasteur to examine the cause of wine spoilage that endangered a major industry in France. Pasteur used microscopy (Figure 8) that he first successfully employed in crystallographic studies in the new biological experiments. In doing so, he discovered that fermentation was spoiling wine because of microorganisms that could be destroyed by controlled heating (38). The technique was named after Pasteur - pasteurization. Pasteur concluded that fermentation was due to living microorganisms rather than to chemical processes. In that regard, he was opposed to the views of the famous chemist Justus von Liebig (1803-1873) who believed that fermentation was due to enzymes (39). A few years after Pasteur's death, the difference in the interpretations of these two famous scientists was resolved when fermentation was found to be produced not only by live microorganisms, but also by enzymes released from dead microorganisms.

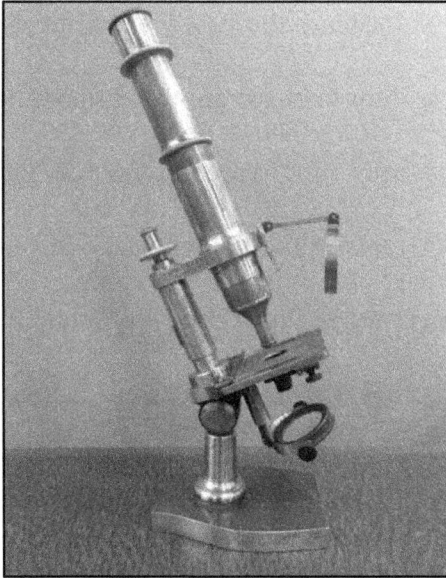

Figure 8. One of Louis Pasteur's microscopes.

This microscope is in the Truman G. Blocker, Jr. History of Medicine Collections at the University of Texas Medical Branch.

Pasteur reasoned early in his scientific endeavors that there could be analogies between fermentation, putrefaction, and infectious disease. In a sense, the idea guided him to examine how microorganisms survived, if those agents caused diseases, and how they could be controlled or prevented.

Anaerobiosis

Leeuwenhoek was the first to observe that certain bacteria survived and multiplied in the absence of air (anaerobiosis), but Pasteur is usually given credit for the discovery because his observations were made under controlled laboratory conditions. It was later discovered that anaerobiosis was due to either fermentation or anaerobic respiration. This 1863 discovery was important because many important bacterial pathogens that cause human diseases were later found to be anaerobic.

Silkworm Infections

After his work on fermentation, an old friend of Pasteur, Professor Jean-Batiste André Dumas at the *Université de Paris,* turned to him to solve another important commercial problem, the decline in the silkworms (the larval form of the domesticated silkworm, *Bombyx mori)* that was wrecking the silk industry in the south of France. Pasteur and four of his best students went to Pont Gisque in Southern France to investigate the problem. After a long period that involved many tedious manipulations and many microscopic observations, Pasteur and his students found that the silkworm disease was caused by two separate kinds of infectious agents (40). Much later, a number of other infectious agents were found to be at fault. In retrospect, the findings were not only important for the beginnings of microbiology, but also because the experimental observations indicated that different pathogens could cause diseases, which had very similar, if not indistinguishable, outward manifestations. Indeed, it was later found that many specific diseases have overlapping pathological and clinical features that may bedevil even the best medical diagnosticians.

Pasteur accurately predicted the evolutionary aspect of virulent microorganisms and their importance in the genesis of human diseases. His following comment on that subject is germane to his subsequent discoveries of vaccines and to many discoveries concerning infectious diseases in the twentieth and early twenty-first centuries.

"Thus, virulence appears in a new light which may be disturbing for the future of humanity unless nature, in its long evolution, has already had the occasions to produce all possible contagious diseases—a very unlikely assumption.

What is a microorganism that is innocuous to man or to a given animal species? It is a living being, which does not possess the capacity to multiply in our body or in the body of the animal. But nothing proves that if the same microorganism should chance to come into contact with some other of the thousands of animal species in the Creation, it might invade it and render it sick. Its virulence might increase by repeated passages through that species, and might eventually affect man or domesticated animals. Thus might be brought about a new virulence and new contagions. I am much inclined to believe that such mechanisms would explain how smallpox, syphilis, plague, yellow fever, etc. have come about in the course of time, and how certain great epidemics appear once in a while."

Vaccines: Chicken Cholera and Sheep Anthrax

Because of his discoveries concerning fermentation and pathogens in invertebrates, Pasteur perceived that pathogens that caused infections in certain vertebrate species could not only be identified but also prevented. As with his earlier research concerning the spoilage of wine and silkworm larva infections, Pasteur was concerned principally with preventing infections that were major threats to public health. He subsequently investigated the cause and prevention of an illness that was decimating domesticated chickens, the chicken cholera (41), anthrax infections in sheep (42), and the dreaded rabies infections in humans (43). His discoveries of vaccines against those pathogens were important milestones in the history of microbiology and immunology and heralded the birth of killed and attenuated immunizations to prevent infectious diseases in humans and other animal species.

In the first of those investigations, in 1880, Pasteur turned an inadvertent experimental error into the production of a vaccine against chicken cholera. It occurred because one of his research associates, Charles Chamberlain, MD (1851-1908), mistakenly left a culture of the chicken cholera pathogen out of the incubator for some days before injecting it into uninfected chickens (26,40). Poultry immunized with that culture survived without any apparent evidence of cholera after being injected with the pathogenic unaltered cholera bacteria. Pasteur reasoned that the pathogens became attenuated after exposure to room temperature and that attenuated pathogens could be used as a vaccine to prevent the disease. This was confirmed in many subsequent experiments in chickens.

Pasteur's next major discovery in preventative vaccines was in a non-human mammal. Pasteur extended earlier observations by the veterinarian Casimir-Joseph Davaine (1812-1882) (44) concerning the morphology of anthrax bacilli and the experimental transmission of anthrax to rabbits. Pasteur discovered that anthrax bacilli lost their virulence but retained their immunogenicity after heating at 42° to 43° C for eight days while the culture preparations were infused with oxygen. However, in the famous successful public trials of the anthrax vaccine that he and his associates carried out in Pouilly-le-Fort in 1881 (37), a variation in a method developed earlier by Jean-Joseph Henri Toussant (1847-1890) (45) was used.

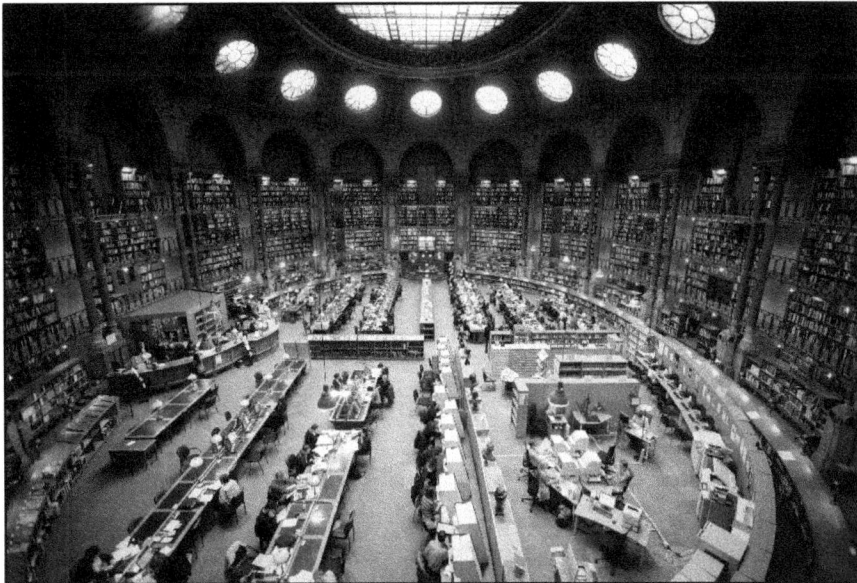

Figure 9. l'Bibliothèque Nationale en Paris.
Where Louis Pasteur's laboratory notebooks are stored.

Pasteur's anthrax experiments were challenged for valid reasons by Pasteur's major rival, the German microbiologist – immunologist Robert Koch, who was famous for his postulates concerning the criteria that a microorganism caused a particular disease (46), the isolation of *Bacillus anthracis* in 1876 (47), and his discovery of the cause of human tuberculosis (*Mycobacterium tuberculosis*) in 1882 (48). Excellent German biologists were unable to create a protective anthrax vaccine by using the published methods. It was dramatic that these two founders of microbiology were at odds about the efficacy of the vaccine. The drama was heightened when they publically debated the issue (49, 50).

Part of the reason for their heated dispute may have emanated from the outcome of the Franco-Prussian War (51), which was humiliating for France. Pasteur was intensely patriotic, and in many ways felt that the success of his research was for the honor of France. So, criticisms by a German scientist were likely not to be well received. However, it should be acknowledged that the German scientists were using the vaccine described in Pasteur's publication, not the one used in the field trials.

Eventually the results of Pasteur's anthrax vaccine experiments were vindicated. But the validity of Koch's question only came to light many years later when it was found that Pasteur's colleagues, Émile Roux and Charles Chamberlain, modified the vaccine by treating anthrax bacilli with the oxidizing agent potassium bichromate (26). That method used in the preparation of the vaccine became known in the 1970s only after Pasteur's laboratory notebooks housed in *l'Bibliotheque Nationale en Paris* (Figure 9) were made available for study.

The First Human Vaccine Created in the Laboratory

Pasteur is probably best appreciated by the general public for creating the first vaccine against the uniformly fatal rabies virus that was a scourge in many parts of the world. The somewhat strange way it was developed is a poignant story.

Inadvertent Laboratory Error Leads to Rabies Vaccine

Pasteur's creation of the rabies vaccine in 1885 was his last original scientific contribution. The development of the vaccine came about two years before the creation of the institute named after him. A way to protect against rabies had been long sought because of the centuries-long fear of the disease that had almost mythical overtones of evil (52). The disease was manifest by prolonged, violent, escalating nervous system symptoms that inevitably led to death. In the minds of many people, it was as though an evil spirit had passed from the bite of a mad dog into its victim.

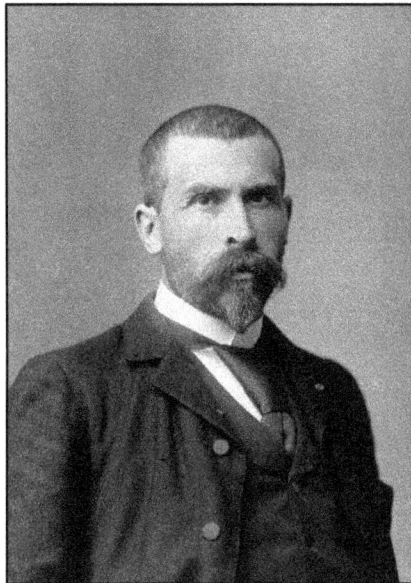

Figure 10. Émile Roux. A colleague of Louis Pasteur was instrumental in developing the anthrax and rabies vaccines and discovered the diphtheria toxin and its antitoxin.

Pasteur reasoned that the disease was due to an infectious agent that disrupted the central nervous system, even though the proposed agent in nervous system tissues could not be seen with optical microscopes used at that time. He and his colleagues

attempted to study the transmission and prevention of the infection by first culturing

spinal cords obtained from experimentally infected animals. When one of Pasteur's

colleagues, Émile Roux, MD (Figure 10), inadvertently left some spinal cords from

rabies-infected animals out of the incubator, the air-dried specimens were found to

be non-pathogenic in experimental animals. The laboratory altered tissue preparation

became the basis for a vaccine against that the human rabies virus. Improved variants

of that vaccine made of human diploid cells, chicken embryo cells, or Vero cells are

currently used to prevent rabies in humans.

Controversy Concerning the Rabies Vaccine

It was disconcerting to learn several decades later that Pasteur first used the vaccine

in an adult who may not have had rabies and in a rabid adult who died before the

vaccine was tested in experimental animals (26). Moreover, when Pasteur's research

assistant, Jacque-Joseph Grancher, MD (1843-1907) who was the head of the

Pediatric clinic at the *Hôpital de Paris pour enfants* (Paris Children's Hospital),

accidentally injected himself with rabies virus, Pasteur convinced Grancher to

receive the vaccine. The injector (Pasteur's nephew, Adrien Loir) and Grancher

received the experimental rabies vaccine without negative effects. Moreover, neither

of them developed rabies. The famous treatment of the nine-year child Joseph

Meister, who was exposed to rabies (Figure 11), came afterwards and before the animal experiments with the vaccine derived from rabbits were completed (26).

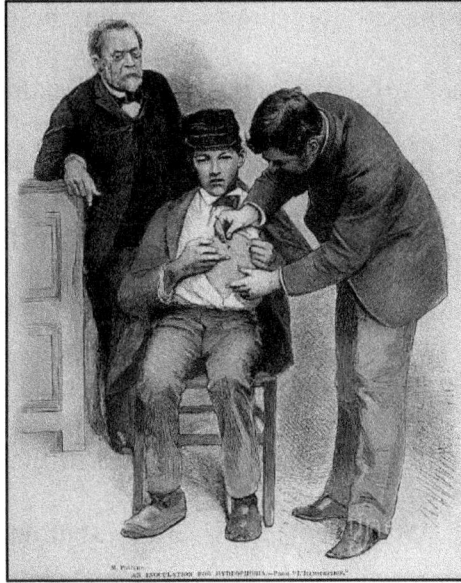

Figure 11. Joseph Meister. The first human treated for rabies with the rabies vaccine developed by Louis Pasteur and his colleagues.

Long afterwards, Pasteur was severely criticized for injecting the rabies vaccine into a human before the experimental animal studies were completed. However, it should be understood that Pasteur did not seek out the child who was severely bitten by a rabid dog. Indeed, the mother of the child upon learning that Pasteur was working on a vaccine to prevent rabies, pleaded incessantly with him to save her child. Pasteur, who was not a physician, first resisted her pleas. He nevertheless knew that rabies was almost always fatal. Furthermore, his preliminary studies suggested that the vaccine was harmless and possibly protective if used soon enough after exposure to the virus. Émile Roux refused to participate in the human experiment because the animal experiments were incomplete. Pasteur supervised the experimental treatment, but the pediatrician, Grancher, administered the injections to the child.

Of course, at this time, stringent guidelines concerning human research would have precluded the use of such an experimental vaccine in humans. Today it would probably take a decade or more to prove the possible efficacy of such a vaccine and to ensure that no long-term adverse reactions might occur. But in the nascent period of experimental immunology, complex regulations of human research were far into the future. Thankfully, the first experimental vaccine used in humans proved to be successful. In that respect, in 1886 Pasteur reported to the *Académie des Sciences française* that 349 of the 350 patients bitten by a rabid animal were saved by the rabies immunization, and no adverse side effects from the vaccine were observed (42).

Why the Rabies Vaccine Succeeded

Fortune favored Pasteur in his rabies vaccine studies because there is a considerable latent period in humans (usually three to eight weeks) between the bite from a rabid animal and the invasion of the brain by the rabies virus. That is because the rabies virus must undergo a number of elaborate steps before infecting the brain (53). First, after the rabies virus enters the host, it replicates in muscle tissue or peripheral nerve cells by binding acetylcholine receptors in those tissues. Pinocytosis (formation of small cytoplasmic vesicles that contain the virus) then occurs, and the rabies virus subsequently enters an endosome (a membrane-bounded compartment) of the cell. Consequently, the five proteins and single strand RNA of the rabies virus are released into the cytoplasm. Then, through an elaborate process in the host cell, new viruses are produced. The newly propagated viruses are released, and when they infect peripheral nerves, they are retrogradely transported to the brain where a fatal encephalitis begins.

An active rabies immunization requires about ten to fourteen days in humans to produce sufficient quantities of circulating antibodies to abolish the rabies virus infection. Thus, if the immunization is given quickly enough, the rabies-infected patient is saved. Although the more modern human diploid cell rabies vaccines are safer and more efficacious, the principles concerning the current rabies vaccine emanate from Pasteur's original studies.

Although some current commentators criticize Pasteur for his somewhat premature use of the rabies vaccine in human volunteers and in individuals who had probably contracted rabies before the experimental animal studies were completed, it should be recalled that rabies was a fearsome, agonizing, uniformly fatal disease. Undoubtedly, Pasteur was torn between the need to complete the experimental animal studies and the possibility that his as yet incompletely tested vaccine might work and save an otherwise condemned victim of rabies. Furthermore, he was handicapped in that there was no way to ascertain whether a bitten individual had rabies until the individual became symptomatic. We now know that if he waited that long in the case of Joseph Meister, who was infected with the rabies virus, the vaccine would have been ineffective, and the bitten child would have died. Finally, it is easy but perhaps not always fair to apply current standards to problems in medical research that occurred well over a century ago. The retrospectroscope is not always accurate.

Pasteur and Serendipity

However, even Pasteur's critics agree that few individuals devoted themselves more avidly to science and applied lessons learned from one experimental field to another than Pasteur. Despite little if any initial training in biology or medicine and a stroke at age 46 that left him partially paralyzed in his right arm and leg, Pasteur made remarkable discoveries in bacteriology, fermentation, infectious disease, and immunology. In that respect, Pasteur commented three years before his discovery of mirror-image populations of organic crystals that "*in the fields of observation, chance favors only the prepared mind*" (26). The three mythical princes of Serendip (hence, serendipity) (54) and the two Jewish slaves in a story by Talmudic Rabbi Yochanan, as related by Rava (55), would have heartedly agreed. The vaccines that Pasteur developed by serendipitous means became the basis for the developments of many other attenuated vaccines that would protect humans and other animals from a host of deadly infectious diseases.

The Complexity of Pasteur's Behavior

There is considerable evidence that Pasteur was a complex individual. On one hand, he was very intelligent, highly imaginative, courageous, versatile, philosophical, tenacious, able to capitalize on inadvertent errors, and dedicated to the control and prevention of serious diseases. His great intelligence was manifest even during his childhood by his love for reading. His courage was manifest during his experiments with the creation of the rabies vaccine when he personally extracted saliva from the mouths of rabid dogs.

He had many reasons to investigate the control and prevention of infectious diseases. Once he ascertained that infections were not generated spontaneously but were spread and reproduced, it was logical for him to predict that ways would be found to retard their spread or prevent their occurrence. That inductive thinking led to his discoveries of attenuated vaccines.

It should be kept in mind that Pasteur's dedication to the control and prevention of infectious diseases very likely was generated by the loss of Louis and Marie Pasteur's daughters, Jeanne at age 9 years (1859) and Cecille at age 13 years (1866) due to what was believed to be typhoid fever. Undoubtedly, those losses further goaded him to develop protective vaccines against microbial pathogens. That would have been not only because of their deaths but also because of the severity and duration of typhoid fever that lasts several weeks (56). Undoubtedly, the agony of the deaths of his two daughters and his inability to help them weighed heavily of his mind and was very likely an impetus to develop vaccines against microbial pathogens.

Although Pasteur would be praised later in his life for his discoveries in microbiology and immunology, his work was often not readily accepted by physicians in France and other countries. In part, the reluctance was because Pasteur was never trained in biology or medicine, and also because his early research had nothing to do with human diseases.

Pasteur became a research chemist in 1843 and by 1854 at age 32; he became *Doyen de la Faculté des sciences* at *l'Université Lille*. At this time, Lille was the center of alcohol manufacture in France.

In 1856, a layman named Bigo, who worked at a factory that made alcohol from sugar beets, visited Pasteur. Bigo's problem was that many of his vats of fermented beer were turning sour. As a result, the beer had to be discarded. Bigo asked Pasteur to find out why this was happening. By using microscopy to analyze samples from the vats, Pasteur found thousands of microbes in the materials from the vats. Pasteur believed that those microorganims caused the putrefaction of the beer. During the next few years he demonstrated that microorganisms also caused the spoilage of milk, wine, and vinegar.

Despite his previous successes in showing the untoward effects of microbes upon commercial products, when he suggested that air-borne microbes could cause disease, he was vilified by many French physicians. One example was a statement in 1860 by Rossignol, a veterinarian at Melun and the editor of *l'Revue vétérinaire*. "*I am afraid that the experiments you quote, M. Pasteur, will turn against you. The world into which you wish to take us is really too fantastic.*"

Even after Pasteur had developed the chicken cholera vaccine, many physicians and veterinarians mocked him. For example, Rossignol wrote the following in 1881.

"Will you have some microbe? There is some everywhere. Microbiolatry is the fashion, it reigns undisputed; it is a doctrine which must not even be discussed, especially when it's Pontiff, the learned Monsieur Pasteur, has pronounced the sacramental words, "I have spoken". The microbe alone is and shall be the characteristic of a disease; that is understood and settled;... the Microbe alone is true, and Pasteur is its prophet."

Rossignol and Professor of Veterinary Medicine Gabriel Colin then challenged Pasteur in 1882 to a public test of his anthrax vaccine (57). The stockbreeders and the veterinarians seemed sure that the test would fail. The President of the Agriculture Society of Melun, Baron de la Rochette, therefore proposed that Pasteur conduct a field trial to prove or disprove the efficacy of the vaccine. The Farmers' Society financed the public test and provided 60 sheep, 10 cattle, and a goat for the experiments that were conducted in *Pouilly-le-Fort* close by Melun, France in May 1882. The results were a resounding success. The vaccinated animals were protected against anthrax. The unvaccinated animals were not. The efficacy of Pasteur's anthrax vaccines silenced most of the critics concerning the importance of the newly emerging fields of microbiology and immunology.

Pasteur's love for his family was poignantly displayed during the midst of the Franco-Prussian War. The war was purposely provoked by the Prussian Chancellor Otto von Bismarck in July 1870 to draw the Southern States of Germany into an alliance with the North German Confederation that was dominated by Prussia (58). The Germans, in contrast to the French, were extensively prepared for combat. Their troops were well trained, well equipped, and transported quickly to the frontlines by rail. The Germans won virtually every battle during the war, whereas the French never stabilized or overturned the conflict.

In January 1871, just a few weeks before the Armistice of that war, the French armies fled in a desperate retreat. The French troops were poorly equipped and disorganized. Many were wounded, poorly clothed, cold, and short of food. Pasteur and his wife Marie set out in a small carriage into the stream of retreating French soldiers to find their son Jean Baptiste (named after the famous scientist Biot), who was a sergeant in the French Army. After several days of fruitlessly searching the bands of dispirited, retreating French troops and nearly wreaking their carriage during their journeys to areas close to the frontlines, they finally found Jean Baptiste sitting despondently in the back of a cart. They were able to bring him to safety and gradually nursed him back to health. But the fear of the near loss of the son was not to be forgotten by the parents.

The French were bitter at the temporary occupation of Paris by the Germans at the end of the conflict, the very high war renumeration and the loss of most of Alsace and part of Lorraine to the Germans. The territorial losses and the humiliation of the defeat were some of the reasons that led to the First World War. Pasteur also never forgot the indignity of the defeat of France by Germany. This was perhaps one reason for the feud between him and the famous German microbiologist Robert Koch

(Figure 12) that centered upon the efficacy of the anthrax vaccine by Pasteur and his colleagues.

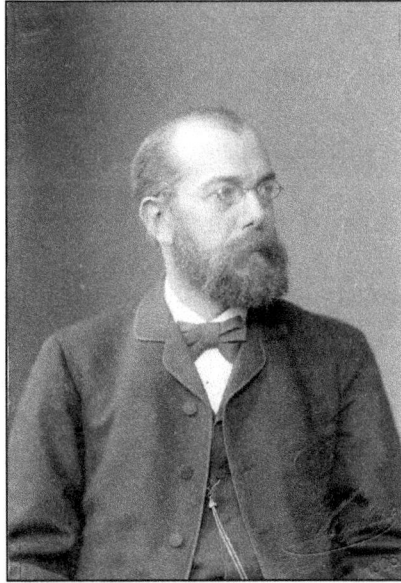

Figure 12. Robert Koch, 1906.
A famous microbiologist who criticized Louis
Pasteur's anthrax vaccine experiments.
(From the Truman G. Blocker, Jr. History of Medicine Collections.)

There was an unfortunate side of Pasteur's persona. He often dealt harshly with some of his closest associates, pointedly did not share his laboratory notebooks with his colleagues, manipulated some research findings to suit his purpose, and displayed considerable anger toward some of his scientific rivals such as Robert Koch when they raised legitimate questions about his research.

His debate with Robert Koch was probably the most famous example of his struggles with other scientists of equal quality. After Pasteur reported the successful vaccination of sheep against anthrax, in 1881 Koch raised grave doubts about the methods and results of the study. At the *Quatrième Congrès Internationale de l' Hygiène et Démographie* in Geneva in 1882, Pasteur delivered a polemic against Koch during his presentation. In turn, Koch publicly ridiculed Pasteur's scientific methods and soon published a detailed critique. Robert Koch maintained that Pasteur failed to reveal the entire nature of the immunogen and the full results of the anthrax vaccine trials. Pasteur vigorously replied to refute the objections.

However, there was another facet of Pasteur that could not be predicted by his fierce competitive nature. That was his compassion for his fellow human beings. That was evident in many ways, but perhaps the most notable was evident in his first use of the rabies vaccine to treat a child bitten by a rabid dog. Pasteur's words are as follows.

"The death of this child appearing to be inevitable, I decided, not without lively and sore anxiety, as may well be believed, to try upon Joseph Meister, the method which I had found constantly successful with dogs. Consequently, sixty hours after the bites, and in the presence of Drs. Vulpian and Grancher, young Meister was inoculated under a fold of skin with half a syringeful of the spinal cord of a rabbit, which had died of rabies. It had been preserved (for) fifteen days in a flask of dry air. In the following days, fresh inoculations were made. I thus made thirteen inoculations. On the last days, I inoculated Joseph Meister with the most virulent virus of rabies."

Pasteur had deep feelings about the pervasive importance of science, and he expressed his views of this important subject on many occasions in private and in public meetings. One quote from one of Pasteur's great admirers, the famous Sir William Osler, was an indication of Pasteur's dedication to science (59). The quote that was used in the preface to René Vallery-Radot's biography of Pasteur (59) is as follows.

"The cultivation of science in its expression is perhaps more necessary to the moral condition than to the material prosperity of a nation."

On the other hand, Pasteur was secretive, exceptionally stubborn, and quick to criticize some of his closest associates for occasional errors. Furthermore, he may have used co-workers at times inappropriately. The development of the anthrax vaccine was a case in point. Pasteur reported that the vaccine was developed by exposing anthrax bacilli to high concentrations of oxygen. But in reality, the vaccine was made by Pasteur's colleagues, Roux and Chamberland, by using carbolic acid. Furthermore, the method was first developed by a French veterinarian, Jean Joseph Henri Toussaint (1847-1890) at the Veterinary School of Toulouse, who also was the first to isolate chicken cholera. Although Pasteur did not initially give Toussaint credit for the first development of the anthrax vaccine, he belatedly recognized him in 1883 by presenting him the Vaillant Prize for his work on anthrax.

Perhaps the most potentially dangerous misuse of his colleagues was during the experiments that led to the development of the rabies vaccine. The injection of the live attenuated vaccine into humans before the experiments in animals were completed was potentially very dangerous. Even if the vaccine seemed safe in experimental animals, it might not have been in humans because of differences in the immune system in mammalian species. Thankfully, the vaccine proved to be safe.

Development of Fellow Scientists

In the last decade of his life, Pasteur stopped conducting research possibly because of the strokes that he sustained, one of which partially paralyzed his right upper and lower extremities. Instead, he took great pains to find private support for the Institute, to develop his colleagues, and to recruit and develop new scientists in the nascent fields of microbiology and immunology. Apropos was the speech that he gave at the opening ceremony of the Institute on November 14, 1888.

"My dear colleagues, maintain the enthusiasm that you showed right from the beginning. At the same time, keep constant vigilance over monitoring operations. Never advance anything that cannot be proved in a simple and decisive manner. Adopt a critical mind. By itself, it can neither encourage ideas nor stimulate anything great. But without it, everything is useless. It always has the last word."

The researchers that he helped to develop included Émile Roux who helped to discover the vaccines, for which Pasteur became famous, co-discovered the cause of diphtheria, developed an antiserum to treat that disease, and became *le Directeur de l'Institut Pasteur en Paris* in 1904.

It was particularly important that Pasteur recruited the soon to be world famous, Russian born biologist Ilya Ilich Metchnikoff (Figure 12) who almost single-handedly discovered the essential roles of phagocytes in defense against infectious

agents and in inflammation and the concept of cellular immunology (6). In 1886,

Metchnikoff was appointed Scientific Director of the Bacteriological Institute in

Odessa. However, despite some successful research he conducted, he resigned

because of a broken promise by the university. He therefore decided to seek a

research position in Western Europe. He first sought out the famous microbiologist

Robert Koch, who headed the *Institut für Hygiene* (Institute of Hygiene) at the

University of Berlin in Germany. But Koch was not interested in Metchnikoff. In

contrast, Pasteur promptly welcomed Metchnikoff to his institute in Paris one year

before his own death.

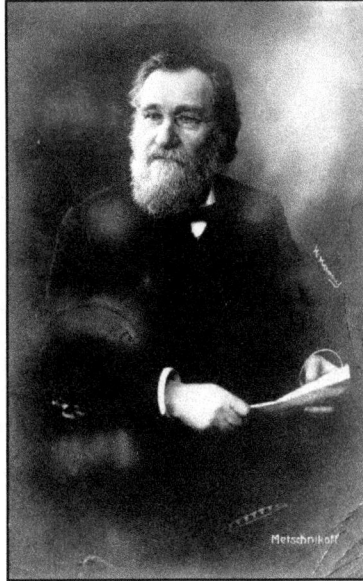

Figure 13. Ilya Ilich Metchnikoff. Discoverer of cellular immunity.
(From the Truman G. Blocker, Jr. History of Medicine Collections.)

Metchnikoff in turn provided the opportunity for the most famous Belgian immunologist, Jules Bordet (Figure 13) to work at the Institute. Bordet went on to discover 1) complement and its binding to antigen-antibody complexes, 2) the complement fixation test, 3) anaphylatoxin, 4) conglutinin, 5) lysozyme in human milk, 6) the formation of thrombin, 7) the participation of platelets in coagulation, and 8) the pathogen that caused whooping cough (7). It is in part to Pasteur's credit that Metchnikoff and Bordet received the prestigious Nobel Prize in Physiology or Medicine in 1908 and 1920, respectively.

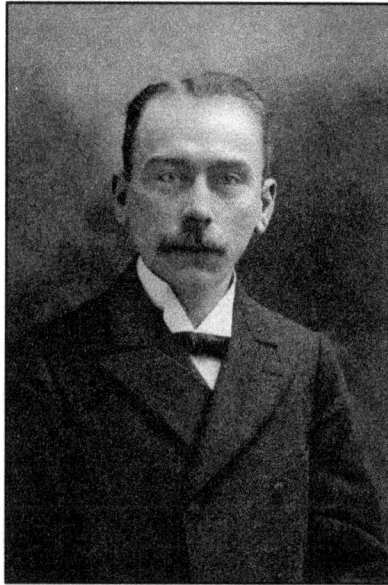

Figure 14. Jules Bordet. This famous immunologist began his first experiments on complement and antibodies in *l'Institut Pasteur en Paris*.

Unfortunately, Pasteur did not receive the Nobel Prize because he died before the award was created. Although he would have richly deserved it, he received many other awards including the Rumford Medal in 1856 for his discovery of the nature of racemic acid and its relations to polarized light, the Montyon Prize in 1859 for experimental physiology from the French Academy of Sciences, the Copley Medal from the Royal Society of London in 1874 for his work on fermentation, the Jecker Prize in 1861, the Alhumbert Prize from the French Academy of Sciences in 1862 for his experimental refutation of spontaneous generation of life, the Leeuwenhoek Medal from the Royal Netherlands Academy of Arts and Sciences, and *The Order of Légion d'Honneur* from the Government of France in 1895.

Genesis of Pasteur's Behavior

A considerable part of Pasteur's behavior may be explained by the inherent features of the brain that control behavior (60). However, it may have been in part because of the somewhat unusual situation that Pasteur encountered during the first phase of his higher education away from his home. He came from a good family who possesed little financial resources. In contrast, the vast majority of his fellow students in higher education were from wealthy families. It is likely that this discrepancy may have created a sense of insecurity in Pasteur and may have discouraged him from becoming close friends with his peers. In that respect, there is historical evidence that Pasteur formed close ties with only a few of his fellow students or colleagues.

Another piece of evidence of Pasteur's reserve toward people who were close to him was his behavior toward his wife, Marie (née Laurent) (1826-1910). Marie was born in Clermont Ferrand, France. She was one of the daughters of the Rector of the Strasbourg Academy. She met Louis when he joined the faculty of the Strasbourg

Academy. At age 23, she married Louis when he was age 26. She was principally responsible for raising their five children and caring for Pasteur later in his life after he was partially crippled by strokes.

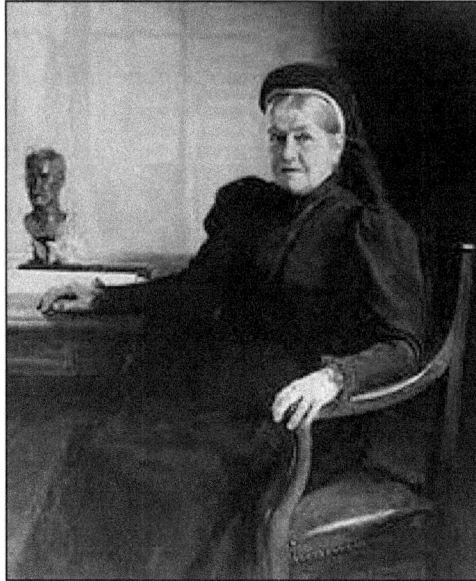

Figure 15. Marie Pasteur, 1899.
Louis Pasteur's wife.

Marie gave Louis abundant help throughout his career, not only as his wife but also as his secretary, literary and artistic assistant, and participant in those experiments concerning organic crystals and the polarization of light. She also grew the silkworms used by Pasteur to demonstrate the causes of the silkworm blight. Marie also helped to care for some of the children who participated in the rabies vaccination experiments. Although Pasteur's assistants spoke fondly of Marie's participation in the research and of her care of their mentor – her husband never publically acknowledged his wife's considerable aid in his professional life. Perhaps that was a reflection of the period in which they lived, in that often women in patriarchal societies were uncommonly recognized for their achievements in professional world including medicine.

How much of his seemingly paradoxical behavior was due to insecurity about his circumstances during his late childhood and early adult life remains to be explored. But one could imagine that Louis never forgot his early childhood even when he became one of the most famous scientists of all time. In that respect, it might be said that one might attempt to deny one's past, but can one forget it?

Thus, Pasteur emerges as one of the most intriguing individuals in the history of science. Given his complex life, perhaps the intrigue concerning his library that was discovered should have been expected.

Chapter 3. Pasteur's Death, Family, and His Library

"There is remedy for all things except death." ~ *Don Quixote,* Miguel de Cervantes

Decline of Pasteur's Health and His Death

Beginning in 1868, Pasteur suffered a series of strokes that gradually incapacitated him. However, because of his dedication to science and his tenacity, he continued to work during those twenty-seven years. The final, fatal stroke occurred on September 28, 1895.

Following his death at age 72, Pasteur was mourned by many millions throughout France and in other countries (17). Indeed, admiration for Pasteur's scientific achievements continues to the present day. His tomb at *l'Institut Pasteur en Paris* remains one of the most frequently visited memorials in France.

Pasteur's Libraries

Pasteur had two libraries. The first was composed of books that he did not write, but did not contain his personal correspondence and certain books and journal articles that dealt with scientific subjects such as microbiology and immunology that were of great interest to him. In 1890, five years before his death, Pasteur asked a Parisian book dealer, Gauthier Villars, to appraise those documents. After the appraisal was completed, Pasteur gave them to the library of *l'Institut Pasteur en Paris*. After 1891, any books or journals that Pasteur obtained were given to *l'Institut*.

The second group of documents was the collection of Pasteur's writings; his letters and scientific articles that appeared in important Western European journals, other writings that he collected, and his laboratory notebooks. Pasteur insisted that the contents of the laboratory notebooks would never be revealed. Much of Pasteur's correspondence and his laboratory notebooks were given to *l'Bibliothèque nationale de France* in 1964 by Pasteur's grandson, Joseph Louis Pasteur Vallery-Radot, MD (Figure 14). The rest of *la Bibliothèque de Louis Pasteur* is the subject of this book.

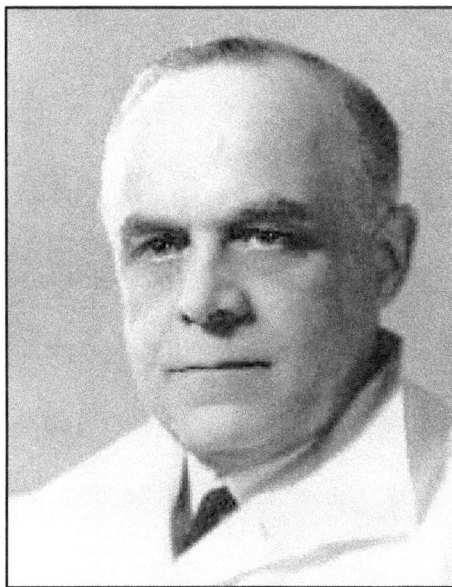

Figure 16. Joseph Louis Pasteur Vallery-Radot. Vallery-Radot played a key role in the fate of the library of his grandfather, Louis Pasteur.

His Personal Library Passes to His Descendants

Pasteur bequeathed his personal library to his wife Marie. She lived for fifteen years after the death of her husband. After her death in 1910 at age 84, *la Bibliothèque de Louis Pasteur* passed to her daughter, Marie Louise (1858-1934) and Marie Louise's husband René Vallery-Radot (1853-1933), who wrote the first biography of Pasteur (52) and who edited many of Pasteur's letters to make them more civil. After the death of René Vallery-Radot in 1933, Louis Pasteur's Library passed to their son, Joseph Louis Pasteur Vallery-Radot, MD (1886-1970) (61) (Timeline 2) who wrote a book about his famous grandfather and who became famous in his own right in the field of medicine.

Joseph Louis Pasteur Vallery-Radot

Pasteur's grandson, Vallery-Radot, was a celebrated French physician during the first half of the twentieth century (62). He was a clinical expert in allergic (62) and renal diseases. By 1927 at age 41, he became *Professeur agrégé de Médecine*. Nine years later, Vallery-Radot was elected to *l'Académie nationale dans la faculté de médecine de Paris*. Two years later (1938), he was appointed as *Professeur dans la faculté de la médecine de Paris*, where he studied allergic and renal diseases and produced a number of important publications concerning the manifestations and treatment of allergic disorders.

Perhaps the most intriguing part of Vallery-Radot's life was during the Second World War when he became *Président du Comité médical de La Résistance française* (Chairman of the Medical Committee of the French Resistance) (63). At the beginning of the German occupation of France, he was briefly detained by the German Gestapo. After his release, Vallery-Radot headed a clandestine operation in *La Résistance française* to medically aid the members of the resistance. For several years, he was pursued by the Gestapo but never apprehended.

Shortly after the end of World War II in 1945, Charles de Gaulle of the Provisional Government of the French Republic appointed Vallery-Radot to head the *Département national de la santé publique* (National Department of Public Health) in France. On October 12, 1944, he was elected to the prestigious *Académie française*. After the end of the Second World War, Vallery-Radot continued his investigations of renal and allergic diseases. His clinical investigations on the therapeutic effects of antihistamines included the use of a neuropsychiatric agent promethazine (Phenergan) in allergic diseases. In 1963, he and his colleagues published an interesting book concerning the manifestations, diagnosis and treatment of allergic diseases (62) that was popular for some time in many countries in Western Europe.

In 1965, President Charles de Gaulle awarded Vallery-Radot the *Croix Grande* for his long, distinguished service to his country. Moreover, for some years, Vallery-Radot served as the president of the institute that was named in honor of his illustrious grandfather and namesake, *l'Institute Pasteur en Paris*. Vallery-Radot died of a heart attack in 1970 at age 84.

Because of the great respect for his deeds to his country and to *l'Institute Pasteur en Paris*, Louis Pasteur Vallery-Radot is still remembered by medical historians and current physicians in France.

La Bibliothèque During World War II

During World War II *la Bibliothèque de Louis Pasteur* was potentially endangered because of the German occupation of France from 1940 until 1945. Furthermore, the danger was intensified by the role that Pasteur's grandson, Joseph Louis Pasteur Vallery-Radot, played during that perilous period.

German Occupation of France During World War II

Following the defeat of France by Germany in June 1940, the *Wehrmacht* permanently occupied the northern and western regions of France. The southern region, except for the Atlantic coast, was placed under the rule of the French military hero of the First World War, Maréchal Henri Philippe Benoni Joseph Pétain (1856-1951). However, Maréchal Pétain was in charge of the south of France in name only. He and his chief associate, the former Prime Minister of France, Pierre Laval (1883-1945), were subordinate to the Germans. At that same time, Italian troops occupied several Departments along the French-Italian borders. German military forces occupied the rest of France and built a large number of powerful highly fortified fortresses, smaller concrete bunkers, and V1 rocket launchers along the entire Atlantic Coast of France to decimate England and to defend against the threat of an invasion by the Allied forces from the sea.

During the occupation, the French were forced to support 300,000 German troops in their country. In that respect, the Germans seized about twenty percent of the French food production as well as many other materials and products. Consequently, shortages in foods and other necessities were common throughout France during the German occupation.

Vallery-Radot found himself in a dire situation because of the German occupation and his important role in *La Résistance française* (55). According to published accounts after his death, his activities in directing the medical support for *La Résistance* were essential to its mission.

Fate of the Library during World War II

During the War, Vallery-Radot's grandfather's library was endangered. Since most of the Nazis had little respect for the French or French scientists, they might have burned the books and papers if they had found them, as they had done with thousands of books during their rise to power during the 1930s. However, there were a number of reasons why the Germans did not desecrate *l'Institut Pasteur* where the *la Bibliothèque de Louis Pasteur* may have been stored. First, as the French were being defeated, their government declared Paris to be an "open city". Therefore, there was very little damage to the Paris by bombers or artillery. Thus, there was virtually no armed combat in the city. That was in stark contrast to the fate of Warsaw, London, and Berlin during the Second World War. The second reason was that the Germans sought collaboration from the French citizens. Any desecration of *l'Institut Pasteur* would have inflamed the passions of the French and surely would have led to a massive revolt of the French citizens against the German occupiers. In that respect, members of *l'Institut* continued to produce certain pharmaceutical agents, antisera, and vaccines against a number of infectious agents including the rabies virus.

However, despite many efforts, it remains unknown how Vallery-Radot protected his grandfather's library. Regardless of how he accomplished the task, at the end of the Second World War, *la Bibliothèque de Louis Pasteur* was intact and undamaged.

Chapter 4. Break-up of *La Bibliothèque*

"The library is the temple of learning, and learning has liberated more people than all the wars in history." ~ Carl T. Rowan

France After the Second World War

Following the end of Second World War and for some years thereafter, most of Western Europe remained decimated. Several million died in that region of typhus in the last year of the war and during the next few years. Basic transportation and other essential industries were badly damaged. France was hard hit during the post-war period because of the prolonged occupation by the German military forces and the battles that occurred throughout most of France after the Allied invasion on June 6, 1944. Because of the protracted combat, most of the agricultural, manufacturing and transportation facilities in France were wrecked or greatly damaged.

The repair of the French economy was slow for the first few years of the post-war period because of the many disruptions in the infrastructure of the nation and the death of 1.3 million French soldiers and nearly three million other casualties during the war. How many suffered permanently from the stress of war among the military and civilian populations is unknown but was likely very high. Because of a paucity of many commodities, rationing of food and other goods continued in France for some years after the Second World War.

In parallel with the economic problems, most of the French academic institutions including the medical schools were slowly reconstructed (64). But *l'Institut Pasteur* as well as certain other institutions of higher learning in France were fortunate to receive considerable financial assistance from the Rockefeller Foundation in order to maintain their staff and upgrade their equipment (65).

The reconstruction of all of these enterprises quickened with advent of the Marshall Plan (the European Recovery Program) in 1948 (66). During the four years of the Marshall Plan, 13 billion United States dollars for economic and technical aid was given to help the recovery of the European countries that had joined in the Organization for European Economic Co-operation. France was one of the principal recipients of funds that provided industrial equipment, foodstuffs, and raw materials that were required to sustain and rebuild the French economy during the three years that the Marshall Plan operated. It is thus understandable that many previously middle to upper class families struggled to regain their pre-war status during the first few decades after the war.

Dr. Vallery-Radot's Life After World War II

In all likelihood, Vallery-Radot and his wife found themselves in difficult financial straits because of the Second World War and its aftermath. He was not paid for his work in the French Resistance. Furthermore, Vallery-Radot's many responsibilities as *Chef du Service de la Santé Publique*, his service in the Constitutional Council from 1959 until 1965 and the High Military Court in 1962, and his work in founding certain important medical research institutions and conducting research after the war may have further curtailed his ability to regain his previous financial standing.

However, the reasons for Vallery-Radot's decision to sell large parts of his grandfather's library were never revealed. In addition to the suggested financial problems, his declining health may have also played a role in the decision to sell the library of his famous grandfather. That suggestion is more tenable since Vallery-Radot and his wife had no children and there were no other living relatives on Pasteur's side of the family. Therefore, after the death of Joseph Louis Pasteur Vallery-Radot and his wife, *la Bibliothèque de Louis Pasteur* would either be given to *l'Institut Pasteur*, *l'Bibliothèque nationale de France*, or sold to wealthy book collectors directly or through an appropriate bookstore in France.

Louis Pasteur's Library is Broken Up

La Bibliothèque de Louis Pasteur, which had been carefully preserved by his descendants for six decades, would now be broken up (Timeline 2) and would come into the hands of a diverse group of very interesting people. They included: 1) a prominent, wealthy American electrical engineer, inventor, historian, book collector; 2) a physician who served in the United States Army during the Second World War and afterwards became a psychiatrist ad became deeply interested in the history of psychoanalysis; 3) a humanist who became the president of a large American state university system and the founder of one of the most extensive historical collections in the United States; 4) an outstanding American radiologist who became interested in the history of medicine by reading to his nearly blind physician - father; and 5) a famous American trauma surgeon who eventually became the president of a major medical school and became immersed in a study of the history of medicine.

The fate of *la Bibliothèque de Louis Pasteur* could have been presented in a temporal fashion, but it is more appropriate to first describe how the fate of one part of Louis Pasteur's Library became known and why that eventually led us to track the circuitous pathways of the rest of those historically important documents.

Chapter 5. First Encounter with *La Bibliothèque*

"Books are the mirrors of men." ~ Anonymous

Piecing together the story of *la Bibliothèque de Louis Pasteur* was like working a jigsaw puzzle. You first find one piece of the puzzle and then you try to discover a second piece that matches the contours of the first piece. And the process continues until the entire picture is reconstructed. The analogy is, however, imperfect, because for some time key pieces were missing from the board. In time, however, they were discovered and much, if not all, of the puzzle was completed (1). What follows is the first piece of the puzzle.

Truman Graves Blocker, Jr.: Part of the Library Comes to Galveston

In 1977, Armond S. Goldman, MD was Professor at the University of Texas Medical Branch at Galveston, Texas. In contrast to most who enter in academic medicine, he joined the faculty of the medical school from which he had graduated. Consequently, he knew many members of the faculty at the school in which he was educated, including its immediate past president, Truman Graves Blocker, Jr., MD (1909-1984) (Figure 17).

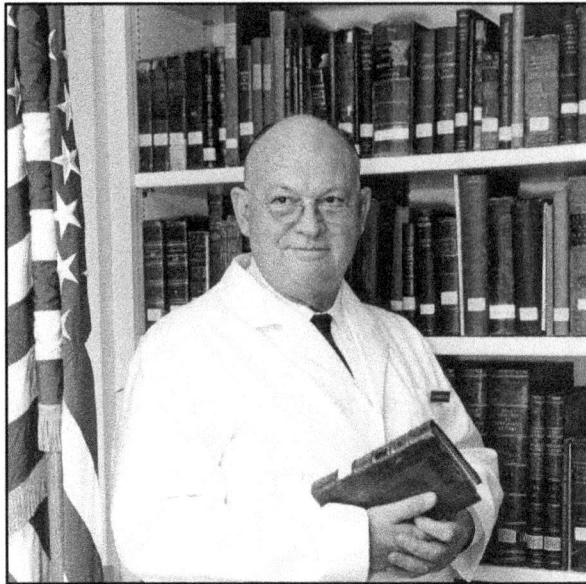

Figure 17. Truman Graves Blocker, Jr. This first President of the University of Texas Medical Branch obtained an important part of *la Bibliothèque de Louis Pasteur* for the University of Texas Medical Branch.

Blocker's Formative Years

Blocker was already a legend at the school that he had led. His life before and after entering the profession of medicine was germane to this story because it indicates how he rose to fame and how he became intrigued with the history of medicine. He was born in West Point, Mississippi on April 17, 1909. Soon afterwards, his family moved to Sherman, Texas, located on the border between Texas and Arkansas. Before then, his father, Truman Graves Blocker, was a school teacher and a salesman in a cotton goods/burlap store in West Point, Mississippi. After moving to Sherman, Truman's father became a salesman for Morgan Hamilton Bag and Bagging Company. In addition, he very soon became a civic leader in the community. He was chosen to be the Head of Stewards of the Methodist Church and Chairman of the

Board of the Young Men's Christian Association.

The Blocker family had several chickens, a cow, and a "fine horse and buggy." When Truman Blocker was 7 years old, his job was to milk the cow every day and deliver the milk to their neighbors. However, his father and an uncle, J. Paul Smith, encouraged the younger Truman's interest in science. Moreover, Truman's mother, Mary Ann Johnson Blocker, prophesized that when Truman grew up, he would become a famous surgeon. Her prophecy was correct.

Medical Training

After graduating from high school, Blocker went to Austin College in Central Texas, where he prepared to apply for medical school. He was subsequently admitted to University of Texas Medical Branch at Galveston, Texas in 1929. That was an unusual period, because it was the start of the Great Depression in the United States. Truman was a very lively student and sometimes got into trouble because of his mischievous behavior. On the other hand, he displayed a genuine interest in many of the medical sciences and worked well with the patients who were assigned to him.

After he was awarded the doctoral degree in medicine from the University of Texas Medical Branch in 1933, Blocker interned at the Graduate Hospital of the University of Pennsylvania in Philadelphia. Afterwards, he spent a year in a surgical residency at the University of Texas Medical Branch. Immediately thereafter, Blocker became an Instructor in Surgery at Columbia Presbyterian Hospital in New York City.

First Phase of Blocker's Academic Life

In 1936, Blocker returned to the medical school in Galveston, Texas as an Assistant Professor of Surgery. During first year as a member of the faculty at the medical school in Galveston, he spent two hour each week giving lectures in surgical pathology and thirty-two hours per week during the fall and spring semesters teaching medical students in the anatomy, pathology, and biochemistry laboratories. During those times, he also performed surgical procedures, conducted some clinical research, published some articles, served on some of the medical school committees, and was frequently on-call for the emergency room.

Blocker's Military Service

Once the United States was drawn into the Second World War in December 1941, Blocker promptly volunteered to serve as a military physician. From 1942 to 1946, he was a military surgeon first with the United States Air Force and then with the United States Army. Blocker rose rapidly in the ranks and was promoted to Colonel and became Chief of Plastic Surgery and then of the Chief of Surgery at the Wakefield General Hospital in Indiana. When he left the Army in 1946, he received the Legion of Merit for his dedicated service and leadership. He continued to serve as a Consultant to the Surgeon General of the United States. Following the reactivation of the United States Army 807th General Hospital in 1956, Blocker was promoted to Brigadier General.

Return to Academic Life and The Texas City Disaster

At the end of his full-time military service, Blocker returned to the University of Texas Medical Branch as the Director of Post-Graduate Education and Professor and Chief of the newly formed Division of Plastic and Maxillofacial Surgery. His medical knowledge, surgical skills, and administrative leadership were soon severely put to the test.

On April 16, 1947 the deadliest industrial catastrophe in United States history, the Texas City Disaster, occurred (67). That morning, a fire began aboard the *SS Grandcamp*, which carried about 2,300 tons of ammonium nitrate. A chain reaction ensued that demolished a nearby vessel, the *SS High Flyer*, that also carried ammonium nitrate, destroyed a third ship, the *SS William B. Keene*, ignited many nearby fuel depots and refineries and obliterated many adjacent homes. About 600 people were killed. Some 3,000 persons were injured – many with severe burns.

Drawing upon his experiences in the military and his natural leadership abilities, at the insistence of the Dean of the school, Blocker mobilized the medical and surgical facilities at the Medical Branch, took charge of the evacuation of the injured victims, and supervised and participated directly in the medical and surgical care of those trauma cases. Students and other trainees depending upon their level of training contributed significantly to the efforts. Some were rescuers, stretcher-bearers, gave first aid, or helped to administer intravenous fluids, blood transfusions, intramuscular medications, immunizations, or surgical care.

He and his wife, Virginia Blocker, MD (1913-2005), later published an extensive medical review of the Texas City Disaster (68). For their research concerning trauma and burns, both of them received the prestigious Harvey Allen Distinguished Service Award from the American Burn Association in 1971.

Rise to Presidency of the Medical School

In 1951, Blocker became the Acting Medical Director of the John Sealy Hospital, and in 1953, he was appointed as the Dean of the Medical Faculty. Afterwards he declined to serve in higher administrative positions because he preferred direct participation in clinical care, teaching, and research.

But because of his outstanding leadership in the institution over many years, Blocker was drafted to chair the Department of Surgery in 1960. Because of his leadership abilities, he subsequently became the Executive Director and Dean and then was appointed in 1967 to be the first President of the University of Texas Medical Branch.

During his seven-year presidency of the Medical Branch, Blocker guided the development of patient care, medical education, and medical research. At that time, all of the academic activities at the University of Texas Medical Branch flourished. Furthermore, he was the driving force for the creation of a clinical science building, a renal dialysis center, the Marine Biomedical Institute, the famous Shriners Burns Institute for Children, the Moody Medical Library, and the Institute of Medical Humanities at the University of Texas Medical Branch.

Blocker's Devotions

Truman Blocker dedicated most of his professional life to build the academic institution and to improve the humanitarian as well as the clinical and scientific aspects of the enterprise. He did so by personally investing in the development of his students and colleagues. In that respect, he had a phenomenal understanding of the lives and professional activities of the members of his faculty.

He was also intensely loyal to his colleagues. One of the major examples came about when the University of Texas System Board of Regents threatened in the early 1970s to dismiss Joseph White, MD, the Vice President for Academic Affairs and Dean of Medicine, and James Thompson, MD, the Chair of the Department of Surgery. Blocker informed the members of the System Board of Regents if that occurred, he would resign immediately. The Regents accordingly withdrew the threat and his colleagues continued to do their excellent work in their same capacities at the Medical Branch.

Blocker's last three major enterprises, the Shriners Burns Institute for Children, the Moody Medical Library, and the Institute of Medical Humanities at the Medical Branch were outgrowths of his pioneering work in the care of patients with burn trauma on the one hand and his great interest in medical history on the other. In a sense, the two came together because he realized that to create new enterprises that one had to thoroughly understand both the misconceptions as well as the successes that occurred in the past.

Blocker's Mentor in Medical History: Chauncey Leake

Blocker's love for medical history developed principally after the Second World War when he encountered and came under the influence of Chauncey Depew Leake, PhD (1896 -1978) (Figure 16) (69). Chauncey Leake's father's ancestors were most likely from Lincolnshire and Nottingham region of England.

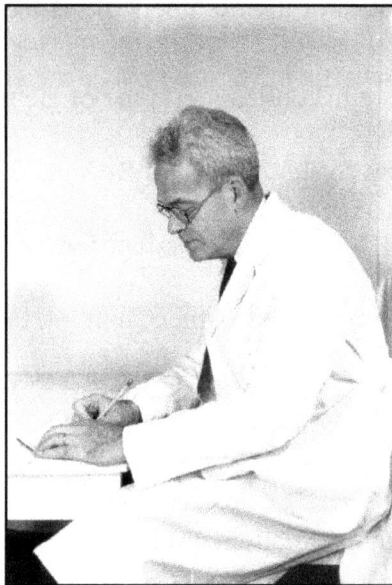

Figure 18. Chauncey Depew Leake.
Dean of the University of Texas Medical Branch at Galveston (1942-1955).
Encouraged Blocker's interest in medical history.

Leake was born in Elizabeth, New Jersey in 1896. His father, Frank W. Leake, was a coal shipper for the Central Railroad of New Jersey. Members of his mother's family were German craftsmen. During his childhood, Leake became enamored by the writings of Mark Twain, Rudyard Kipling, and Robert Louis Stevenson and the fictional exploits of Sherlock Holmes. In high school, he was an excellent student but also participated on the football and track teams and was manager of the baseball team. Leake continued to be a leader for the rest of his days.

In 1917, Leake graduated with a Baccalaureate from Princeton University after majoring in philosophy, chemistry, and biology. Shortly after the United States entered the First World War in April 1917, he enlisted in the New Jersey National Guard and was placed in a machine gun training group. However, because of his high intelligence and his previous studies in the sciences of biology and chemistry, he was reassigned to the Chemical Warfare Service in 1918 to develop counter-measures against poisonous war gases. As the First World War drew to a close by November 1918, Leake's research concerning poison gases ceased. However, he remained in the United States Army to investigate the pharmacological effects of morphine, since that was one of the principal drugs that could relieve the pain inflicted by war wounds.

After Leake left the United States Army, he thought about becoming a physician, but instead he entered the graduate school program at the University of Wisconsin. In that program, Leake studied physiology and pharmacology. He subsequently received a Master's Degree in 1920 and a Doctor in Philosophy in Pharmacology in 1925. Afterwards, Leake taught pharmacology and physiology for the next several years at the University of Wisconsin. In addition, during those years and before then, Leake read extensively about the history of science and medicine. Because of his success in academic work, in 1928 he was asked to establish the Department of Pharmacology at the University of California in San Francisco. He accepted that position and also became the Senior Lecturer in the History and Philosophy of Medicine at that institution.

Leake was a quintessential Renaissance man: a master pharmacologist, humanist, ethicist, and historian (69). Leake made many significant contributions to the field of medical pharmacology at the University of California in San Francisco including the metabolic action of anesthetics and narcotics, the regulation of the production of red blood cells, the biochemistry of the brain and other parts of the central nervous system, and the treatment of leprosy. Furthermore, Leake formulated a conceptual basis of pharmacology as a medical-scientific discipline.

In 1942, Leake became the Dean of the University of Texas Medical Branch (the chief administrative office at that time). He may have been the first non-physician to lead a medical school. It was a somewhat difficult time to take over the reins of leadership at that medical school, because it was during the first year of the participation of the United States in the Second World War and also at a time that the school was in disarray because the prior leadership had been inadequate and there was a threat to discredit the school. But during those difficult years, Leake inspired the members of the faculty and the students to attain excellence and thus create in his own words, a community of scholars. In that spirit, Leake convinced Blocker to rejoin the University of Texas Medical Branch after the Second World War ended

Blocker was intrigued by Leake's vision of an institution that brought medical sciences together with art, history, and ethics of medicine. Over the next decade,

Leake encouraged Blocker to develop the famous burn care center and to help build strong programs in medical ethics and history. As the programs in medical ethics and history grew, rare books and journals that dealt with the history of European and American medicine were acquired.

Blocker Learns of Potential Sale of Pasteur's Library

As President Emeritus during 1974 -1984, Blocker's academic energies and ambitions, which had been imbued by Leake, were undiminished. Blocker continued to teach at the bedside of patients, lecture to medical students and surgical residents, participate in special academic committees, and conduct symposia in medical humanities and history. He also encouraged groups of medical students to study medical history and ethics and to integrate that information with their knowledge of the science and art of medicine. On many days during those years, he took great pleasure in studying the lives and accomplishments of the surgeons of the Renaissance period including Ambroise Paré, who was exceptionally skillful in surgical techniques particularly concerning cleansing and sealing battlefield wounds with natural antiseptic preparations used centuries before by Roman physicians, and who reintroduced the use of ligatures first used by Galen to close bleeding blood vessels. Paré also invented ocular prosthetics, described phantom pain, now known as causalgia, and aided in improving obstetrical techniques.

Blocker took great pleasure in examining many valuable documents housed in the History of Medicine Collections of the library that pertained to surgical care and other subjects that deeply interested him. He was also instrumental in obtaining funds to purchase rare books concerning the history of medicine for that collection. In that spirit, he was convinced that the future of medicine lay not only in increasing medical technology but also in training physicians to become enlightened in the art, ethics, and history of medicine.

Goldman Sees Part of the Louis Pasteur Collection

Perhaps the culmination of Blocker's last activity, the purchase of rare books and other documents in the history of medicine for the History of Medicine Collections, came about in 1977. In early April of that year, Blocker called Goldman on the telephone to "volunteer" for a special assignment.

"Goldman, Truman Blocker here. How in the hell are you? Still experimenting with human milk? How is your wonderful wife Barbara and how about those excellent children? Let me see now - your oldest is Lynn. And how is the oldest boy, David? And Daniel is just as bright. I see that they are ace students. Three children to be in medical school - you must tell me about Paul and Robert when we have time. You and that beautiful, intelligent wife of yours, Barb, should be very proud of all of them."

Blocker, or as he was fondly called "The Tank" or "The General" (but not to his face) because of his frame, his fame in the United States Army Medical Corps, and his enormous academic stature, maintained a mental dossier on many members of the faculty, community physicians, politicians and other key people. It was a matter of a moment for Blocker to put any one at ease and be eager to serve him well and hence do service to the medical school. Goldman soon arrived at his office and found the "General" to be in an exceptionally good mood. The conversation between Blocker and Goldman went something like this:

"Armond, I have a favor to ask you. Pasteur's Library is going on the auction block very soon. Yes, that's right. It is wonderful. It's Louis Pasteur's Library – well, at least half of it. Armond, I would appreciate if you would go to Frisco and check it out for me."

"Dr. Blocker, I'll be glad to do that, but I know nothing about rare books."

"That's not the reason that I am asking you to go. Damn it, Goldman, I need an immunologist to check it out, and you're one of the few on this campus who fits the bill. I need someone who appreciates the history of immunology and microbiology – someone who understands the importance of the pioneers in those fields – someone I know and trust."

With that explanation, Goldman saluted (mentally, that is) and told him he would be glad to help. As Blocker knew beforehand, Goldman was to give a paper at the conjoined meetings of the American Pediatric Society and Society for Pediatric Research in San Francisco in two weeks. Blocker activated the speakerphone and instructed his secretary to call Jeremy Norman in San Francisco. In a few minutes, he had Norman on the line.

"Jeremy. Good to talk with you. How's the weather in 'Frisco'? That's good. Have

you eaten in that good seafood restaurant by the wharves lately? Yes, that's right -

the one that we were at a month ago. Be my guest the next time I'm in town. Look,

Jeremy, I'm sending one of my immunologists to visit you in two weeks and look at

the Louis Pasteur Collection. Will that be reasonable? It will? Very good! Shall we

set it up for (Goldman mouthed a time) – say for that Thursday afternoon? Very good!

At about one o'clock it will be.

Jeremy, as I've told you before, that collection belongs here at the Medical Branch,

so don't sell it until we have a chance to buy it. By the way, the doctor who will visit

you is Armond Goldman. You got that? Jeremy, thank you again. Jeremy, you're a

good guy and a credit to your father. Call me if you have any questions. Otherwise,

I'll call you after Goldman's visit."

Goldman asked Blocker how the Pasteur collection came to reside in a bookstore in
San Francisco. Blocker told the story and later it became even clearer as to how it
came to be.

Haskell Field Norman and the Pasteur Collection

Around 1970 Jeremy Norman's father, Haskell Field Norman, MD (1915-1996)
(Figure 17), a psychiatrist in San Francisco, California learned that approximately
200 items from *la Bibliothèque de Louis Pasteur* were to be sold by the Parisian book
dealer François Chamonal, who had obtained them from Pasteur's descendants.
Norman purchased the collection and brought it to his home in San Francisco.

Norman was a noted psychiatrist and a bibliophile. He was born on July 24, 1915 in Lynn, Massachusetts and was educated at the Boston Latin School and Johns Hopkins University. After doing postgraduate work at Harvard University and working for several years in the shoe industry, he entered medical school at St. Louis University. He was an excellent student and graduated first in his class.

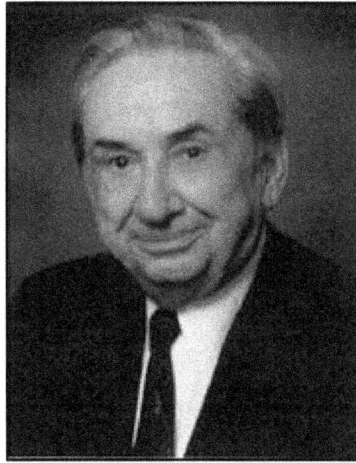

Figure 19. Haskell Field Norman. This American psychiatrist obtained a significant part of *la Bibliothèque de Louis Pasteur* and later passed it to his son, Jeremy.

Norman was subsequently drafted into the United States Army Medical Corps. During his service, he completed a psychiatric residency at the Langley Porter Clinic and Letterman General Hospital in San Francisco. After his military service was completed, he began a psychiatric practice in San Francisco and became a trainer in psychoanalysis at the San Francisco Psychoanalytic Institute.

Norman developed a deep interest in medical history and historical medical texts, particularly in respect to psychiatric diseases. He began collecting important historical medical documents in 1953 when he obtained a first edition of Sigmund Freud's *Die Traumdeutung* (The Dream Interpretation). Since Norman was a psychiatrist, it was natural that his first collections concerned the history of that particular medical specialty. Afterwards Norman broadened his interests in other aspects of medical history and began collecting important historical texts in other aspects of medicine (70). That was further evidenced just before his death when he authored the book, *One Hundred Books Famous in Medicine* (71) that included the Aldine Editions of Hippocrates, the profuse writings of Aelius Galenus better known as Galen: Pedanius Dioscorides' *De Materia Medica*; and Ketham's *Fasciculus medicinae* (six independent and quite different medieval medical treatises).

Norman's son, Jeremy Michael Norman (Figure 18), shared his father's love for medical history and book collecting, but not his zeal for the practice of medicine. Jeremy Norman began his career in the history of science, medicine and technology in 1964 when he was nineteen. He worked as an assistant to the packing clerk at John Howell-Books, the Dickensian bookshop located near Union Square in San Francisco for five and a half years while he was studying at the University of California at Berkeley.

Jeremy Norman received his Bachelor of Arts degree from the University of California, Berkeley in 1969, with a major in history and an emphasis on science. Two years later (1971), he opened the bookstore, Jeremy Norman Rare Books and Manuscripts on Sutter Street in San Francisco. At that time, Dr. Norman gave his

Louis Pasteur Collection to Jeremy (Timeline 2), since he felt that the collection, though obviously very valuable, did not fit the major theme of his library, the field of psychiatry. Six years later (1977), Jeremy Norman decided to sell the Pasteur collection that was given to him by his father. Blocker was one of the first to be informed, since Jeremy Norman had previously sold other valuable historical medical documents to him.

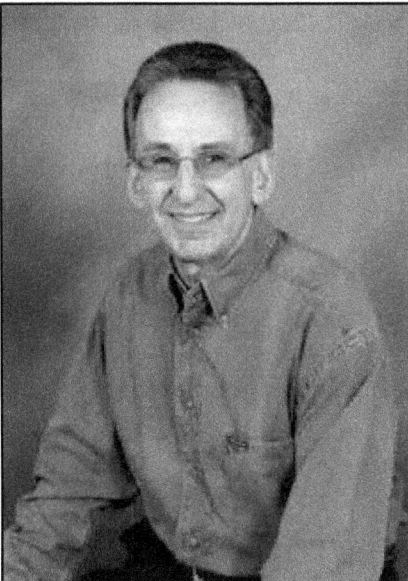

Figure 20. Jeremy Michael Norman. This son of Dr. Norman was the book dealer who sold part of *la Bibliothèque de Louis Pasteur* to the University of Texas Medical Branch.

Blocker continued his conversation with Goldman. *"Goldman, see my secretary on your way out. She will redo your airplane and hotel reservations. They need to be upgraded to first class. And don't worry about the tab. This one is on me."*

In fact, the costs came out of his own pocket, not the University's. Goldman accordingly went to San Francisco and after the morning session of the Pediatric Society meeting was over, he made his way on the Thursday afternoon in question to

Jeremy Norman Rare Books and Manuscripts located at 442 Post Street. He rang the doorbell and within moments, a gentleman immaculately dressed in what in a way resembled Victorian garb, greeted him cordially. "*Dr. Goldman, I presume. I am Jeremy Norman. I am so pleased that you have come in Dr. Blocker's stead to examine the Louis Pasteur Collection.*"

Mr. Norman guided Goldman to a large rectangular room that seemed to belong to another age. All around were medical memorabilia. It reeked of history – of learning – of the bygone days when the basis of modern medicine was being established. The Louis Pasteur Collection was laid out on several tables. There were 154 textbooks, all of Pasteur's published papers, offprints, prints, manuscripts, autographed letters, unpublished autographed manuscripts, letters by Pasteur and statues and busts of him. There were letters from Pasteur requesting funds from the French Government for research and support of his institute, ground-breaking articles by Pasteur including his disproof of spontaneous generation of life, Metchnikoff's famous book concerning immunity in infectious diseases (72), a first edition of Alfred Donné's *Cours de Microscopie* (73) that reproduced the first photomicrographs, the papers by Charles Darwin (1809-1882) and Alfred Russel Wallace (1823-1913) on biological evolution due to natural selection that were presented in 1858 to the Royal Society of Biology (74), a first edition of Darwin's *On the Origin of Species by Natural Selection, or the Preservation of Favoured Races in the Struggle for Life* (36), research papers annotated by Pasteur, 30 papers by Pasteur's German rival Robert

Koch (75), 82 papers by the mercurial, brilliant, pioneering immunologist and immunochemist Paul Ehrlich (6), and many other priceless items.

Occasionally Norman seemingly would magically appear to tend to Goldman, who was oblivious to time. Norman would comment on an item from the collection that Goldman was examining. Norman would wax eloquently and then vanish as ethereally as he came. After more than ten hours engrossed in a treasure of medical history – into the very beginnings of medical microbiology and immunology, Goldman realized that night had fallen. Goldman was embarrassed. He apologized to Norman for his insensitivity, but Norman laughed lightly and said he was happy to see that the Pasteur Collection was so greatly appreciated. And what microbiologist, immunologist, or medical historian would not have been elated with the opportunity to view a significant part of *la Bibliothèque de Louis Pasteur*?

The next morning Goldman flew back to Galveston. On Monday when he arrived at his office, there was a message to see Blocker that afternoon.

Blocker greeted him enthusiastically. "*Goldman, Jeremy tells me that you did a great job. I'm proud of you. Jeremy was impressed. He tells me that you were up until the wee hours of the morning. Tell me about it.*"

Goldman related that the collection was priceless. Any physician, immunologist, or microbiologist would be elated to have the Louis Pasteur Collection in their institution. Blocker made a few telephone calls. Sometime later, The Moody Foundation in Galveston, Texas purchased the Collection for the medical library that bears its name and the Collection was placed on permanent loan with the Truman G.

Blocker History of Medicine Collections. In 1999, the Moody Foundation gave the

Louis Pasteur Collection to the University of Texas Medical Branch at Galveston

where it is housed in the History of Medicine Collections (Figure 21) that is named

in honor of the past president and one of the truly illustrious figures at the University

of Texas Medical Branch, Dr. Truman Graves Blocker, Jr.

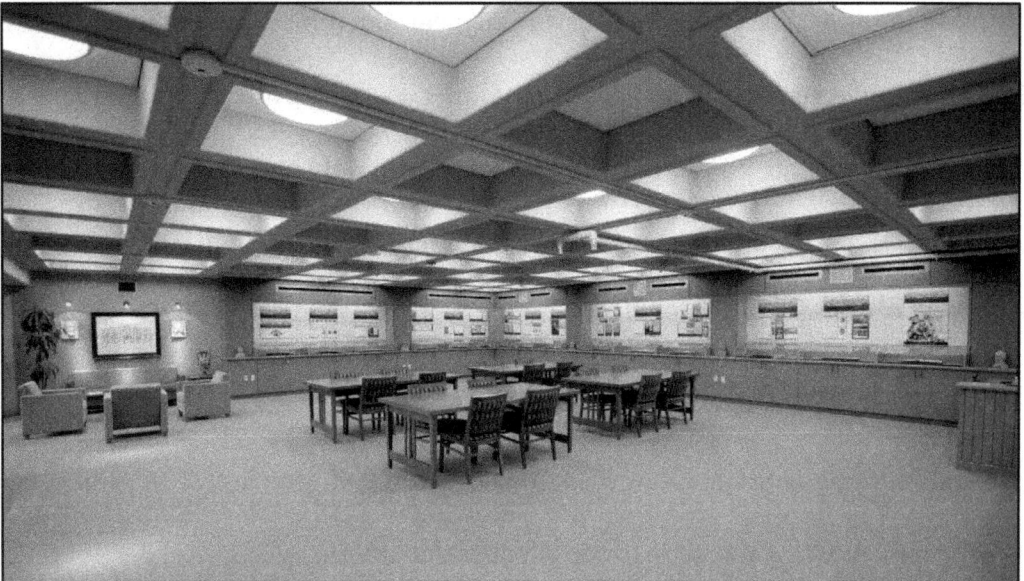

Figure 21. Truman Graves Blocker, Jr. History of Medicine Collections.

Chapter 6. The Mystery Deepens

"The possession of knowledge does not kill the sense of wonder and mystery. There is always more mystery." ~ Anaïs Nin

Discovery of Another Part of the Library

Another major part of *la Bibliothèque de Louis Pasteur* was discovered while we were researching Pasteur's scientific achievements. Dr. Gerald L. Geison reported in his book, *The Private Science of Louis Pasteur* (26), that the bulk of Pasteur's research including his original laboratory notebooks were housed in the *Bibliothèque nationale de France*. Geison also stated that other segments of *la Bibliothèque de Louis Pasteur* could be found in numerous locations outside of France including the Wellcome Institute in London and also in what had been part of the Burndy Library of the History of Science and Technology once housed in Norwalk, Connecticut. These documents were later relocated to the Huntington Library in San Marino, California (Figure 20). It was then revealed by Philip Weimerskirch, Associate Director of the Burndy Library during 1982-1989, how this important part of the *la Bibliothèque de Louis Pasteur* came to the Huntington Library.

Bern Dibner

The trans-Atlantic journey of the part of *la Bibliothèque de Louis Pasteur* that came to the Huntington Library began with Bern Dibner (1897–1988) (Figure 21).

Formative Years

Dibner was a famous electrical engineer, industrialist, and historian of science and technology. He was born in Lisianka, near Kiev, in the Ukraine in 1897 (76). Anti-Semitism had been festering in Western Russia and other parts of the Pale of Settlement for many decades. A large-scale wave of anti-Jewish mob attacks known as pogroms swept the Ukraine in 1881, after Jews were wrongly blamed for the assassination of Tsar Alexander II. There were pogroms in 166 Ukrainian towns. Thousands of Jewish homes were destroyed, many families reduced to extreme poverty, large numbers of men, women, and children were injured, and some were killed. A conference was convened at the Ministry of Interior of Russia, and on May 15, 1882 the so-called Temporary Regulations were introduced that stayed in effect for more than thirty years.

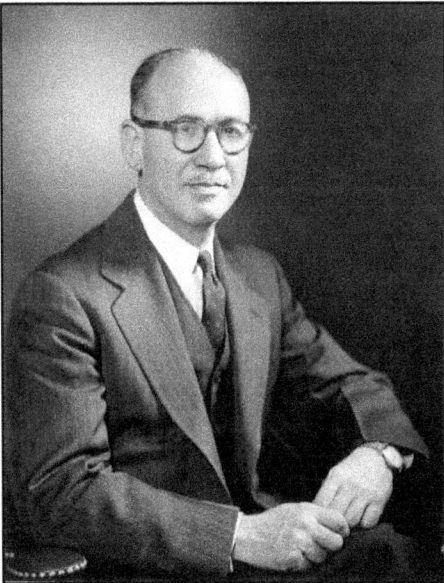

Figure 22. Bern Dibner.

This experimental electrical engineer and history of science collector obtained part of *la Bibliothèque de Louis Pasteur* that resides in the Huntington Library.

These continued restrictions progressively limited where Jews could live, when they could transact business, where they could be educated, and the occupations they might seek within the Pale of Settlement of the Tsarist Russian Empire. In time, Jews were barred from voting in certain communities, and restrictions were placed on the numbers of Jews who could practice medicine or law. Restrictions escalated and a particularly large pogrom that broke out in 1903 in Kishinev, the then capital of the province of Bessarabia. This and the start of the Russo-Japanese War may have convinced the Dibner family along with many other hundreds of thousands of Jews to immigrate to the United States in 1904. The Dibners settled in the Lower East Side of New York City (77). Bern became a naturalized citizen of the United States in 1913.

Bern, the youngest of the children in the family, began attending the newly founded Hebrew Technical Institute at age seven. There he learned alongside other immigrant boys to become technicians. Bern often spoke of the good fortune to have had an excellent headmaster, Edgar Starr Barney (1861-1938), whom Dibner credited with his entrance into the engineering profession (76). As he grew older, he attended this school during the day and in the evenings went to lectures at the Cooper Union. During his teen-age years, he became proficient in both the arts and sciences, but eventually decided to become an electrical engineer (78).

Military Service

In addition to this schooling, Dibner was trained in the Air Force/Army Air Corps in Plattsburgh, New York to investigate the effectiveness of aerial bombing. He would later serve in the European Theatre during the Second World War. His chief duty was to study firsthand the effectiveness of bombing on buildings, bridges, and cities. For these efforts, Dibner attained the rank of Lieutenant Colonel and was awarded the Bronze Star and two Battle Stars (76).

Higher Education

When he returned from the military after World War I, Dibner worked as an electrical maintenance technician in the printing field (77). An accident at this job provided him with a $650.00 worker's compensation settlement, which was enough money for him to attend the Polytechnic Institute of Brooklyn. In 1921, he graduated *summa cum laude* and class valedictorian with a degree in electrical engineering from the institute (78). That same year he traveled to Germany to attempt to develop an import business. However, the effort was not successful.

Engineer, Inventor, and Historian of Science

Upon his return to the United States, Dibner went to work for the Adirondack Power and Light Company in Schenectady, New York, and then with the Electric Bond and Share Company. At that time, the Electric Bond and Share Company was involved with the transmission of electricity in Cuba (77). By 1923, Dibner attempted to unify many small power plants that were scattered across the island, typically in places such as sugar plantations. Each had its own generators and transmission lines and it seemed impossible to form a grid from the different sized cables and connectors. It was crucial to have connections that tied one electrical conductor to the end of another and attach any branch circuitry together. His solution was to invent a universal connector. But he took it one further step - his connector did not require soldering or welding. In addition, it provided a more flexible joint, which could withstand the force of hurricane winds to which Cuba often experienced (77).

Since the Electric Bond and Share Company had no interest in his invention, Dibner patented the design. It was the beginning of a series of patents that launched his career. A year later, he partnered with his brother-in-law to establish the Burndy Engineering Company. The name of the company was a play on his name, Bern D. As his early patents stated, he was named Abraham Bernard Dibner, but his later patents revealed that he had legally changed his name to Bern Dibner by which his friends and colleagues knew him. He developed two-dozen patents over the course of his career including those for terminals and connectors, which eliminated awkward positions for linemen working on power poles. These inventions formed the basis of a very successful company that provided the means for him to begin collecting valuable historical books (77).

Dibner's Preoccupation with Leonardo da Vinci

The Burndy Engineering Company was first located at 43th Street and Fifth Avenue, only a block away from the New York Public Library. It is not known whether the availability of a world of library materials so close at hand, or whether he retained the interest in the arts he had in his younger years stimulated his interest in history of Leonardo da Vinci.

It is documented that around 1929 Dibner read a book that changed him forever. The book, Stuart Chase's *Men and Machines*, detailed the engineering works of Leonardo da Vinci, whom Chase called "*perhaps the most astonishing genius born of woman, and certainly the greatest engineer that ever lived*" (77).

Dibner was astonished to learn from the book that da Vinci created over two-dozen important inventions or theories in the 15th century (79). They included:

1. *The postulation of a theory of wave motion, and the undulating motion of light and heat.*

2. *The laws of a lever moving on an inclined plane, and the formulae for the volume of water needed to fill canals.*

3. *Tides are due to the pull of the sun.*

4. *Invention of the barometer and projection of the thermometer.*

5. *Use of cams, worms, ratchets, sprockets and chains.*

6. *Invention of a stone cutting saw.*

7. *Designs of a steamboat, steam pumps, and steam cannon.*

8. *Designs of buoys, diving apparatus, and the first life preserver.*

Dibner was quoted as saying, "*I was irritated by the preposterous technical feats attributed to Leonardo. I said to myself, somebody really hoodwinked this Chase fellow. So I set out to read everything I could on da Vinci to find out what his real contributions were.*"

Begins to Collect Historical Documents Concerning Science

Subsequently, Dibner devoted himself to the study of da Vinci and his works and his passion for the arts and sciences that paralleled Dibner's to determine whether Chase was correct. He began his collection of da Vinci materials, and by 1936, he decided to take a year's "industrial sabbatical" with his wife, Barbara, and their son, David. The family toured Rome, Vinci in Tuscany (the birthplace of da Vinci), and Florence in search of historical documents concerning da Vinci and other historical scientists, inventors, and artists. After visiting the Italian cities, the Dibners went to Switzerland where Bern attended the University of Zürich and studied history and the Renaissance culture. He focused on the art, science and technology of the period. By learning the Italian language to study more closely da Vinci's works in the libraries and universities on the continent, he found that Stuart Chase had been correct (77).

With this chance encounter with da Vinci's works and his studies abroad, Dibner had been thoroughly introduced to what he called *"the fathomless world of books."* He noted (78):

"...books were the symbol of thought, of innovation, experimentation, discovery. Books prompted the conclusion that our immediate universe was not geocentric.... Books were the medium that proposed that man was one with nature. From books we learned the universal law of gravitation, the structural order of the elements, of electricity, the earth's magnetism, the microscopic nature of bacteria, and the relativistic complexity of subatomic particles and energy. Is it any wonder that a serious wanderer thru this wondrous world gathers such evidence of science and moves to preserve it and hold it for further scholarship and investigation?"

Expands His Collections of Historical Books

While on his European trip, Dibner began buying important old books concerning the history of science and technology. Indeed, he became one of the leading collectors of those valuable documents during the first half of the twentieth century. He did so by forging relationships with the European book dealers and that created important bonds of mutual interest that lasted the remainder of his life.

The First World War and the economic depression in the 1930s took a great toll on European book dealers. It was a buyer's market. For example, in as late as 1925, a copy of Newton's *Principia* published in the 1690s and bound in vellum could be purchased for $22.00. So, for a man with Dibner's means, the sky was the limit (77).

Not long after his return to the United States, from 1940-41, Dibner enrolled as a special student at Columbia University in New York City and undertook a formal study of the history of science. He even studied Latin to better understand the subjects that interested him (76).

Dibner Creates Extensive Libraries

While his intellectual pursuits continued, the Burndy Engineering Company flourished. In 1933, it was moved to Bruckner Boulevard in the Bronx. It was there that the books he purchased formed a library in Dibner's office. Soon, they overflowed into the corridors and eventually to the offices of his associates. The Burndy Library was officially chartered in 1941 as a nonprofit educational institution. That was five years before Harvard instituted the first history of science course in the United States (77).

In 1951, the company moved to an 11-acre site in Norwalk, Connecticut. There the books were housed more appropriately in different conference rooms with names such as the Newton, Einstein and Leonardo Rooms. Twenty-five thousand volumes were eventually collected, and space once again became a premium - necessitating a building of their own. The Burndy Library building, designed by Robert Rogus, opened in 1964 on the Company's grounds (80). It was:

"...a prime source for scholars and researchers who are preparing treatises and monographs on some aspect of the history of science. It shelves also contain a wealth of biographical reference material and "runs" up to three centuries of philosophical

transactions of leading scientific and technical societies outside the U.S. for the benefit of graduate students, researchers and scholars. The registry book in the main reading room contains the names of many students, engineers, prominent scientists, and educators from all over the world."

This library was home to an amazing array of works by many of the greatest minds in science - Isaac Newton, Thomas Edison, Robert Boyle, Robert Hooke, Albertus Magnus, Thomas Aquinas, Charles Darwin, and William Harvey - along with the largest single collection of the Library of Alessandro Volta, the Italian physicist who invented the electrical battery. The library also served as a museum where important historical documents such as a page of the Gutenberg Bible, a manuscript sheet from Darwin's *On the Origin of Species By Means of Natural Selection, or the Preservation of Favoured Races in the Struggle for Life,* and an array of electrical generators, telescopes, vacuum tubes and other scientific equipment were displayed (80).

Dibner Writes Treatises Concerning the History of Science

Dibner's Library mounted many exhibitions and produced publications, often authored by Dibner himself. The most famous of these is *Heralds of Science* published in 1955. In this work, he described the two hundred books that he considered to be the most important ones in the development of science. Each entry for these classic works contains a brief account for the reason of the title's importance along with many illustrations. It is a text still used by bibliographers and booksellers as a reference tool.

Dibner's Gifts to Academic Institutions

As a man who believed he received much in his life, Dibner also believed he should share what he had been able to acquire with other libraries and institutions of learning. Brandeis University was among the first to receive a gift from the Burndy Library when in 1959, he gave the entire collection of the famous Italian mathematician and physicist Vito Volterra, some twenty-four thousand books and pamphlets, and a part of his Leonardo da Vinci collection of more than a thousand items. Dibner also contributed a significant amount of his Library to Harvard, Yale and Wesleyan Universities, the Polytechnic University in Brooklyn and the University of Bridgeport, Connecticut. Perhaps his greatest contribution was to the nation that provided a home for him and his family through a donation of eleven thousand volumes to the Smithsonian Institution in Washington, DC, during the Bicentennial Year, 1976. This gift included the two hundred titles that formed the basis of *Heralds of Science*, along with three hundred and twenty incunabula - the largest collection of books published before 1501 - and all remaining manuscripts from the Burndy Library (78).

Not only was Dibner generous with his books, his philanthropy extended to endowing the Bern and Barbara Chair at Brandeis University and a gift to the Polytechnic University that made possible the construction of the Bern Dibner Library there. In

the late 1980s, he established a curatorship for Einstein Archives and a chair for
Research and Teaching in the History of Science at the Hebrew University in
Jerusalem. He was also a major supporter of the library of the Technion University
in Israel (78).

For his many efforts, Dibner was awarded many accolades. He received the Sarton
Medal from the History of Science Society and the Smithson Gold Medal from the
Smithsonian Institution. The Polytechnic Institute conferred upon him an Honorary
Doctor of Engineering and honorary professorship (76).

After "re-collecting" many of the works he had previously donated, another of
Dibner's great endeavors was to establish the Dibner Institute for the History of
Science and Technology, a consortium in the greater Boston area in 1987, the year
prior to his death. The Institute and Burndy Library were later housed at the
Massachusetts Institute of Technology in 1992 and was hailed as "one of the world's
premiere collections of historical scientific books, manuscripts, instruments and
works of art".

When the hosting arrangement with the Massachusetts Institute of Technology was
to expire in 2007, the Dibner family conducted a national search for other locations
for the Library to ensure its continued use by researchers. In 2006, David Dibner, the
son of Bern and Barbara Dibner, along with other family members decided to move
the sixty-seven thousand volumes comprising the Burndy Library to the Huntington

Library in San Marino, California. That is where the collection of Pasteur materials now resides (81).

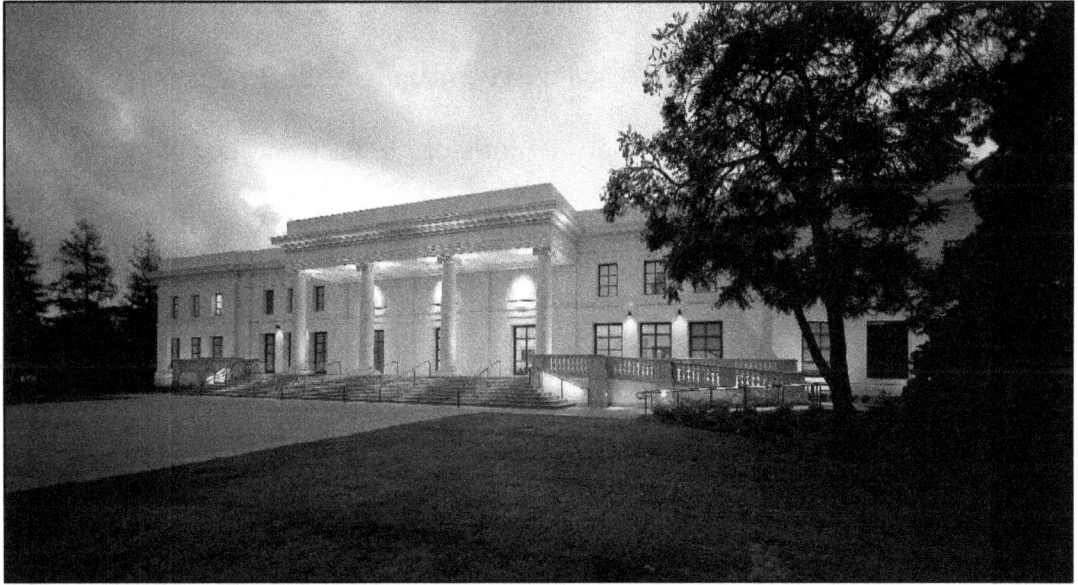

Figure 23. Huntington Library in San Marino, California.

Dibner Acquires an Important Part of Pasteur's Library

Dibner delighted in collecting the great works and contributions of the world's most important scientists. He was also determined to share them with the public. Therefore, it was not a surprise that in 1970 when he learned that part of *la Bibliothèque de Louis Pasteur* was about to be sold by Alain Brieux, a Parisian antiquarian book dealer (*Librarie Brieux*, 48 Rue Jacob). Here were texts and other items that had not been donated to the *Bibliotheque nationale* or kept by the *Institut Pasteur* but had been retained by Pasteur's descendants. Dibner, as he had before, befriended the book dealer and was thus positioned to acquire the documents.

Over a span of some years Alain Brieux and Pasteur's grandson, Joseph Louis Pasteur Vallery-Radot, became closely bonded. According to Brieux, Vallery-Radot entrusted his grandfather's works to him (Timeline 2). Brieux began creating an extensive catalog and marked each cataloged item as authentic. Brieux was asked not to sell the collection until after Vallery-Radot's death. Pasteur's last blood relative, Vallery-Radot, died in October 1970. Sometime, in the early 1970s, Brieux finished the work that Vallery-Radot had requested. Brieux noted in a brief preface note, "*It is not without emotion that I begin the description of the deposit that was entrusted to me*" (82).

Dibner's purchase of the documents from the Louis Pasteur collection included many autographed manuscripts, texts, notebooks, and images. Those items came to the Burndy Library over a period of time. When Brieux visited Dibner in 1985, he brought another precious cargo of Pasteur's documents packed in a plain suitcase. The visit was somewhat of a gamble for Brieux for he did not know whether Dibner would purchase the items. While Brieux was being hosted for lunch by the Burndy Library's Assistant Director, Philip Weimerskirch, Dibner perused the collection and decided to buy it. Shortly after the trip to visit Dibner, Brieux died and took with him this part of the story of *la Bibliothèque de Louis Pasteur* (83).

Chapter 7. Further Insights. The Radiologist

"The true mystery of the world is the visible, not the invisible." ~ Oscar Wilde

After the research concerning *la Bibliothèque de Louis Pasteur* seemed complete, two other parts were discovered.

Part of Pasteur's Library comes to the Reynolds Historical Library

Information concerning Pasteur's famous experiments with anthrax vaccination in sheep was found that helped to trace the trans-Atlantic journey of an additional part of *la Bibliothèque de Louis Pasteur*. Those documents were found in the Reynolds Historical Library at the University of Alabama at Birmingham (Figure 22). Michael Flannery, Curator of the Reynolds Historical Library at the University of Alabama at Birmingham, noted that the library possesses seventeen letters written between Pasteur and his protégé Louis Thuillier (1856-1883) concerning the experimental trials with the anthrax vaccine in sheep and a few other items that were from *la Bibliothèque de Louis Pasteur*. The donor of those important historical documents was Dr. Lawrence E. Reynolds (1889-1961) (Figure 23). Reynolds gave those documents from *la Bibliothèque de Louis Pasteur* along with some 5000 volumes on other subjects in the history of medicine to the University of Alabama in 1955 (84) (Timeline 2).

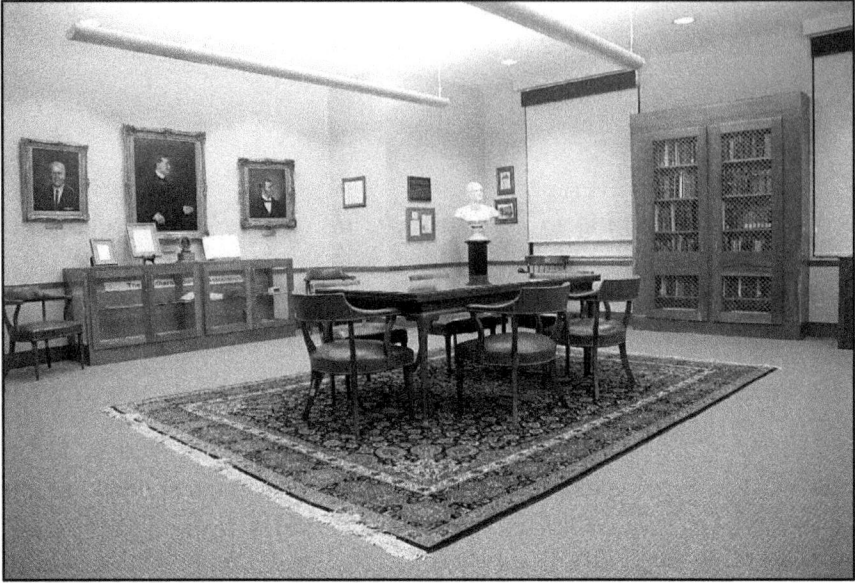

Figure 24. Reynolds Historical Library
at the University of Alabama at Birmingham.

The Story of Dr. Lawrence Reynolds

The story of Lawrence Reynolds, MD (1889-1961) is intriguing and germane to this story. His life began in a rural community in Alabama and ended after he became a nationally acclaimed radiologist.

He acquired important correspondence to and from Pasteur and gave them with many other important medical historical documents to the University of Alabama in Birmingham.

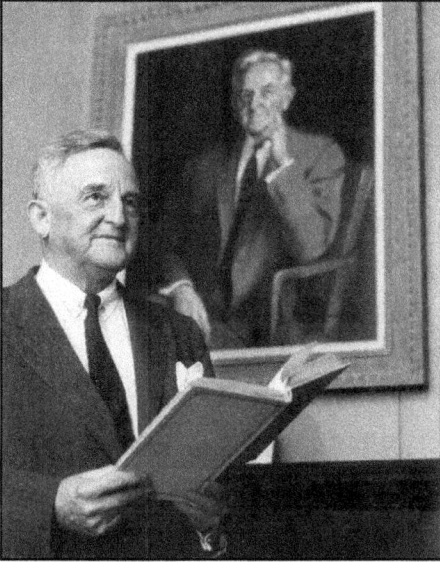

Figure 25. Lawrence Reynolds.

An outstanding American radiologist, bibliophile and the founder of Reynolds Historical Library obtained the part of *la Bibliothèque* that resides there.

His Childhood and Professional Education

Lawrence Reynolds was born in 1889 in the small community of Skipperville, Alabama. His grandfather, father, and two of his older brothers were physicians. As a youth, Reynolds or one of his two brothers accompanied his father, Dr. Robert Davis Reynolds, Sr., a partially blind rural physician, on house calls to his patients by horse and buggy. En route and back from the calls, Reynolds recalled that for four years he frequently read medical treatises to his blind father including some stories concerning the history of medicine and Sir William Osler's famous book, *The Principles and Practice of Medicine*. In this way, he developed a deep appreciation for medicine and its history.

By age 12, Reynolds had enough knowledge of medicine to assist his father in his medical practice. After finishing public school in the local community, Reynolds went to the University of Alabama at Tuscaloosa, Alabama with the intention of becoming a lawyer. But three years later, he decided to follow the family tradition and became a physician. His experience with his physician father may have been the deciding factor in his decision to embark upon a career in medicine.

After receiving a Bachelor of Science Degree from the University of Alabama in 1912, Reynolds attended the Medical School at Johns Hopkins University in Baltimore, Maryland. During his studies in medical school, he was undoubtedly strongly influenced by lectures concerning the history of medicine given by noted physicians in the field. He graduated from the Johns Hopkins University Medical School in 1916.

Service in World War I

Reynolds enlisted to be a military physician and served in that capacity from 1917 through 1919 in the American Army in France during the First World War. Captain Reynolds first assisted in the selection of X-ray equipment that was to be sent to the American Military Hospital in Paris. That was of interest when one considers that the X-ray had been discovered only a few decades before in 1895 by the German physicist Dr. Wilhelm Conrad Röntgen at the *Universität of Würzburg* in Germany by using experimental discharge cathode ray tubes invented around 1875 by the English physicist William Crookes. In that respect, only one year before the start of the First World War, William D. Coolidge invented an X-ray tube with an improved cathode that allowed for more intense visualization of deep-seated anatomy. Thus, the clinical applications of radiology quickly became a reality in civilian and military life. That discovery undoubtedly impressed Reynolds and was most likely one of the reasons that he eventually chose to be a radiologist.

After helping to complete the installation of the X-ray equipment at the American Military Hospital in Paris, Reynolds was assigned to the American Ambulance Service of the US Medical Corps that was located close to the front lines of the military conflict between the Allied forces and the German troops in France. Reynolds and his medical colleagues undoubtedly administered to many wounded and dying soldiers on the front lines during that terrible conflict.

Reynolds Becomes a Radiologist

Once the war was over in 1918, Reynolds returned to Johns Hopkins University to study radiology. Afterwards, he became an Instructor in Radiology in that medical school. Reynolds was then asked to direct the radiology department of the Peter Bent Brigham Hospital in Boston, and he became the Chief of the Department of Radiology at the Medical School of Harvard University.

At Harvard, Reynolds became friends with the noted neurosurgeon Dr. Harvey Cushing, who further stimulated Reynolds' interest in the history of medicine. It is unclear whether Reynolds and Cushing met during the First World War when Cushing was the Senior Consultant in Neurological Surgery for the American Expeditionary Forces in France on the Western front in northern France in 1918. But he and Cushing were undoubtedly closely associated because of the extensive use of radiology in the diagnosis of cranial neoplasms and other cranial disorders that might require neurosurgery.

Although Reynolds earned only a modest salary when he was at Harvard Medical School, he purchased a first edition of the famous book of anatomy by Andreas Vesalius, *De Humani Corpus Fabrica*, published in 1543. He also further cemented his interest in medical history when he read part of the manuscript prepared by Cushing of the *Biography of Sir William Osler*, one of the most famous physicians of his time and a noted medical historian. As already recounted, that was a reinforcing influence, since he had read Osler's book on medical practice when he was with his father on his house calls.

After his service at Peter Bent Brigham Hospital and Harvard Medical School, Reynolds joined a group of private radiologists in Detroit in 1922 and became Professor of Radiology at Wayne University College of Medicine. Thereafter, he served as a Clinical Professor of Radiology at that medical school.

Because of his achievements in the field of radiology, he was elected President of the American Roentgen Ray Society and of the American College of Radiology. He was also selected to be the editor of one of the leading journals in radiology, The American Journal of Roentgenology and Radium Therapy. He continued to be the editor of that journal for thirty-one years. For his outstanding work in that medical specialty, in 1956, Reynolds received the highest award, the Gold Medal Award, from the Radiological Society of North America.

Reynolds Begins Collecting Medical History Books and Other Documents

Reynolds had a lifetime obsession with the history of medicine. While at Johns Hopkins University in Baltimore, Maryland, Reynolds began his medical history collection that ultimately comprised of over 10,000 books, letters, and pamphlets (84). A significant part of Reynolds' collection was obtained from the rare book dealer, Henry Schuman, located in New York City (85). The collection, as previously mentioned, is housed in the University of Alabama in Birmingham.

As previously mentioned, most of Reynolds' collection was purchased from Henry Schuman Rare Books Limited located in New York City. However, it is unclear where Reynolds purchased the important letters between Pasteur and Thuillier concerning the experimental trials with the anthrax vaccine in sheep. That is important, since those letters may have been the first part of *la Bibliothèque de Louis Pasteur* that was sold by Vallery-Radot (Timeline 2).

Chapter 8. Final Link in the Chain

"No 'University of the first class' will ever be achieved without a 'library of the first class.'" ~ Harry Huntt Ransom

It was quite unexpected that the final link in the chain of discoveries concerning *la Bibliothèque de Louis Pasteur* would be in a second part of the University of Texas and would involve one of its outstanding leaders, Harry Huntt Ransom, PhD (1908-1976) (Figure 24).

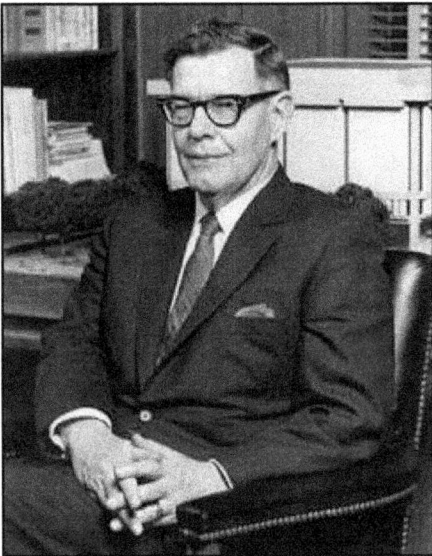

Figure 26. Harry Huntt Ransom.

Past Chancellor of the University of Texas System and creator of The Harry Ransom Humanities Research Center at University of Texas obtained part of *la Bibliothèque* that resides there.

Harry Ransom Humanities Research Center University of Texas

The Harry Ransom Humanities Research Center (Figure 25), originally called the Humanities Research Center when it was formed in 1957 by Ransom (86) at the University of Texas in Austin, Texas, was found to have many important documents from *la Bibliothèque de Louis Pasteur* (Timeline 2). These documents include four autographed manuscripts by Pasteur's son-in-law René Vallery-Radot (1853-1933) of the first published study of Pasteur's life and his work; manuscripts with numerous autographed corrections and additions by Pasteur; books from *la Bibliothèque de Louis Pasteur* with annotations and notes by him; books inscribed to Pasteur, including one from Metchnikoff's lectures on immunity; books by and about Pasteur from his family's libraries; fifty mounted photographs and prints, many with autographed notes by Pasteur relating to the founding of *l'Institut Pasteur*; and a pen-and-ink portrait of Pasteur's close associate, Dr. Émile Roux, signed by the artist and subject.

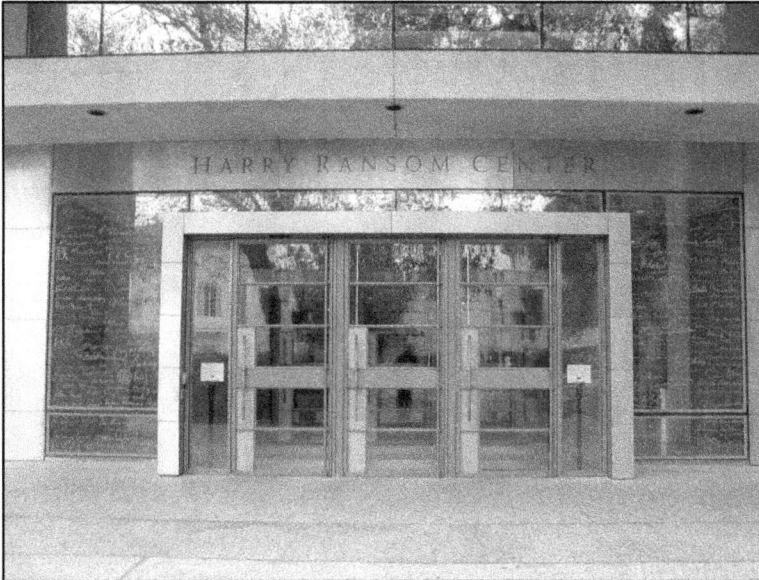

Figure 27. *The Harry Ransom Humanities Research Center.*

How Part of Pasteur's Library Came to the Ransom Center

Margaret Tenney, Head of the Reading Room of The Harry Huntt Ransom Center, related that Ransom (Timeline 2) obtained his portion of *la Bibliothèque de Louis Pasteur* in the late 1960s from Lew David Feldman, the owner of the House of El Dieff in New York City (Timeline 2). How that the proprietor of the House of El Dieff obtained those valuable documents is as yet an unsolved part of the mystery of *la Bibliothèque de Louis Pasteur*.

The Life of Harry Huntt Ransom

Ransom is an intriguing character in the story of the dispersal of *la Bibliothèque de Louis Pasteur*. In that respect, he was the only bibliophile who obtained parts of *la Bibliothèque de Louis Pasteur* who was neither a physician nor a scientist.

Ransom's Early Formative Years

Harry Huntt Ransom was born on November 22, 1908 in Galveston, Texas, where strangely enough, another part of *la Bibliothèque de Louis Pasteur* resides. His parents were Harry Huntt Ransom, Sr., a high school Latin teacher, and Marion Goodwin Ransom. Harry Ransom, Jr. received his early education at a public school in Houston, Texas. After his father's declining health and eventual death, his mother Marion moved the family to Sewanee, Tennessee, where they lived in the Hodgson Hospital where his mother worked. Harry studied at Miss Dubose's Private School, Sewanee, Tennessee, and then at the Sewanee Military Academy. At age 20 (1928) he graduated with a Bachelor of Arts degree from the University of the South at Sewanee.

Higher Education - Start of an Academic Career

Ransom must have been an exceptional student because he was accepted to Harvard University in 1929. After one year at Harvard University, he interrupted his formal education and took a number of different teaching positions. He taught English and journalism at the State Teachers College, Valley City, North Dakota (1930–32; 1933–34) and English and history at Colorado State College, Greeley, Colorado (1934–35).

In 1935, he joined the University of Texas in Austin as an Instructor in English. Ransom then restarted his formal education by entering Yale University. Why he switched from Harvard to Yale was not clear. He completed his studies and obtained a PhD in English at Yale University in 1938. Ransom then spent one year in post-doctoral studies in English literature at the University of London. In 1939, Ransom also founded and served as Director of Research for the International Copyright League in London.

Service in the United States Army Air Force in the Second World War

At the start of the Second World War, Ransom joined the United States Army Air Force as a Second Lieutenant and worked in military editorial intelligence. He was progressively promoted. In 1947, Major Ransom was awarded the Legion of Merit for his excellent military service.

Return to Academic Life - Rise to Chancellor of University of Texas System

After leaving the military, Ransom became Professor at the University of Texas in Austin. His principal research was in the field of copyright law. In that respect, he published a definitive study of the first copyright statute. Ransom also wrote many other articles in scholarly journals and contributed a series of articles about the history of Texas. Because of his academic prowess and his intense interest in education, he was asked to join the Administration of the University of Texas as Assistant Dean of the Graduate School in 1951. In the next decade, Ransom was promoted to Associate Dean in 1953, Dean of the College of Arts and Sciences in 1954, Vice President and Provost in 1957, President in 1960, and Chancellor of the University of Texas System in 1961.

Ransom was dedicated to the development of students at the university and particularly to those who were scholarly inclined. In that regard, as Chancellor of the University of Texas System, he was instrumental in expanding libraries throughout the University of Texas System. But he concentrated principally on developing the main campus of the University System in Austin, Texas.

Establishment of the Harry Ransom Humanities Research Center

Ransom's most lasting contribution was the Harry Ransom Humanities Research

Center with its vast collections of literature, the history of science, iconography, theatre arts, photography, and cartography. In this respect, the library was cited in 1970 in Anthony Hobson's book *Great Libraries* as one of the thirty-two leading libraries in Western Europe and North America (87).

The building of that library and the acquisition of its many precious items needed not only Ransom's vision and tenacity but also considerable financial support that came from millions of dollars garnered from the booming oil industry in Texas. Indeed, the oil flowed to a great extent from oil fields that were located on vast tracts of land that had been given to the University of Texas. Those vast sums and Ransom's brilliance came together at the right place at the right time.

Ransom operated on the assumption that a university library that started in 1883 might aspire by the mid-twentieth century to enter the elite group of older institutions with superior rare books and other manuscript collections. If that came to pass, such a library would attract ambitious faculty members and students at the University and inevitably national and international visitors. That was accomplished by the dint of vigorous support from administrators, regents, legislators, and private benefactors in the State of Texas.

In Ransom's opinion, *"No 'University of the first class' will ever be achieved without a 'library of the first class'."* Ransom believed that it was necessary to build an extraordinary library since students at the University of Texas *"are so far distant from the great concentration of libraries in Chicago and the East Coast."* (85).

Ransom's Legacy as a Scholar and Bibliophile

His active and often successful pursuit of rare books and manuscripts caused him to be known as the *"Great Acquisitor"*. Ransom said to the book dealer, Lew David Feldman, on one occasion the following.

"We do not want to give the impression that Texas is raking in indiscriminately a lot of books simply for the pleasure of raking them in. This plan is carefully calculated to advance scholarship and to give our younger people a laboratory for ideas."

Ransom's intense feelings for libraries and in particular for those that housed rare books were expressed (86) in the following way.

"I am deeply-almost passionately-interested in the printed word. I think that great libraries are something great universities cannot do without. I think no library is great unless it is active and growing...I think the work of university presses, importance of learned periodicals, the role of books, pamphlets, public lectures must be emphasized."

In 1957, Ransom tried to dispel the public's impression of rare books as museum pieces.

"Some of them are...But the real significance of research collections in Texas lies in the vitality they add to modern study" (86).

He amplified on his thoughts of that subject in an address he gave to the Texas Philosophical Society (85).

"Why should Texas not establish here in the capital city...a center for the collection of knowledge, a 'central' for the diffusion of information?...The great urban, regional, and national centers for the collection of knowledge in London, Paris, Dublin, and Edinburgh were begun on an almost pitiable fraction of what this state could spend...Most important of all, young Texans who now are persuaded to leave the state for collections elsewhere might be persuaded by such a research center to stay; and some who have left might be persuaded to come back."

Ransom's definition of rare books included newspapers, pictures, and manuscripts that were very hard to come by. He believed that these materials were essential to the work of young students, scholars, and creative writers. The very valuable collection that he established at the University of Texas reflected his deep respect for rare books and their worth to a wide range of students, scholars, and writers. That is of course exemplified in that part of *la Bibliothèque de Louis Pasteur* that Ransom acquired for the University of Texas.

Chapter 9. What is Gained from Studying *La Bibliothèque?*

"All we know is still infinitely less than all that remains unknown."

~ William Harvey

You might ask why a thorough study of *la Bibliothèque de Louis Pasteur* is important other than to satisfy the compulsion of professional historians and other bibliophiles. As one recent commentator stated, *"little if any insight can be gained by examining the personal libraries of current famous people because the books that are there were written by someone other than the owner of the library"* (88). The writer based his remarks on one library that he encountered - his father-in-law's. However, that point of view does not pertain to the libraries of famous individuals such as Pasteur who lived long before the onset of the current digital age.

Pasteur's Time Compared to the Digital Age

Pasteur is a prime example of the insight that might be gained from a study of the library of a famous individual. In the nineteenth century when Pasteur worked in science and was making many valuable discoveries, the situation was quite different from what we encounter in the digital age. In Pasteur's time, there were no computers, FAX machines, or hand-held digital devices that could be used to transmit or receive images of articles or books. To keep abreast of what he was investigating, Pasteur had to read the books, periodicals, and journals that contained the research reports concerning crystallography, microbiology, and immunology. Thus, early on in his career, Pasteur began collecting the relevant documents in the sciences in which he was interested. Therefore, each book, journal, note, or letter had a personal meaning to him, because they usually impinged upon his thinking and his research.

Books Are the Mirrors of Men

There may be more to it than that. In that respect, a scholar once said that books are the mirrors of men. Indeed, they often reveal more about the writer than verbal conversation alone unearths. Perhaps that also pertains to the books and other documents that a scientist collects. Indeed, they may illuminate what influenced the thinking and approaches to research of the researcher. Modern scholars have been unable to completely explore *la Bibliothèque de Louis Pasteur* because of the uncertainty of the whereabouts of much of its original contents. Indeed, one of the main purposes of this book is to provide those scholars that opportunity.

Although much is known about Pasteur, he remains somewhat of an enigma. Perhaps that is to be expected of genius. However, now that much more of his library has been recovered, there may be more opportunity to further elucidate his complex character.

Indeed, a detailed analysis of Pasteur's Library may well reveal certain aspects of his intellectual development during his early years in research, which previous scientists or thinkers influenced him, and his attitudes toward his colleagues, fellow scientists, and his rivals in the then nascent fields of crystallography, microbiology and immunology. In addition, the absence of certain important scientific reports from one's library may be just as informative. For example, Pasteur apparently had no copies of Gregor Johan Mendel's groundbreaking publication concerning his investigations of the genetics of garden sweet peas (*Pisum sativum*) that Mendel used to elucidate the mathematical pattern of autosomal dominant and recessive inheritance (89). Of course, the same could be said for Mendel and Darwin. In that respect, Darwin was unaware of Mendel's experiments concerning the genetics of garden peas in which he demonstrated the law of independent assortment by examining the color of the peas during a multitude of crossbreeding experiments (89, 90). The inheritance of yellow peas was dominant; that of green peas was recessive.

Curiously enough, Darwin conducted in 1865 similar plant-breeding experiments with snapdragons and published the reports of the experiments a few years after Mendel's report (91). Darwin's experiments were very similar to Mendel's experiments with sweet peas, but Darwin failed to perceive what is now known as Mendelian genetics. Mendel had read a German translation of Darwin's very important book of biological evolution due to natural selection before the publication of his salient article on plant genetics, but apparently, he did not connect Darwin's findings with his own observations. In the case of Pasteur, his seemingly unawareness or disinterest in Mendel may not have made any difference, given his tenacious, single-minded emphasis upon the development of methods to uncover the cause of serious infections and defeat them by developing vaccines to the pathogens. Furthermore, it is doubtful that the discovery of the basic mathematical laws of genetics would have helped Pasteur advance his particular research into microbiology and immunology.

Chapter 10. The Bibliophiles and Pasteur's Library

"Judge a man by his questions rather than his answers." ~ Voltaire

Another unanticipated benefit concerning the curious fate of *la Bibliothèque de Louis Pasteur* was the discovery of the interesting lives of the several bibliophiles who obtained the known segments of that library. Besides their love of medical history, what did these bibliophiles have in common? From what has been pieced together, the following commonalities were found. 1) Three were born of parents of modest means who encouraged their child to attain a higher education (Bern Dibner, Truman Blocker, and Harry Ransom). 2) All were well-educated, highly trained professional men. 3) Three were physicians who became renowned specialists in their fields (Lawrence Reynolds in radiology, Haskell Norman in psychiatry, and Truman Blocker in surgery). 4) All served as officers in the United States Army and three (Harry Ransom, Bern Dibner, and Truman Blocker) received special awards for their service. 5) All received awards from national societies for their scholarly contributions to science, history, or the arts. 6) Two became the principal leader of a major academic institution in the same state (Harry Ransom and Truman Blocker). 7) All established or greatly expanded special libraries. 8) Two (Bern Dibner and Haskell Norman) wrote treatises concerning the history of science or medicine. 9) All were attracted for different reasons to the historical figure of Pasteur. 10) In each case they, or their descendants, made sure that each

segment of *la Bibliothèque de Louis Pasteur* went to an institution that would

protect the works and make them available under appropriate supervision to

scholars in the history of medicine.

Even more basic to their personas, each of them wished to journey back in time - to

discover not only how their own specialties in medicine, physics, or the humanities

developed and determine who were the brilliant people responsible for those

developments - but also to transcend their primary interests and reach out to other

beginnings of our modern-day society. In that respect, they were endowed with

curiosity, with a desire to go beyond the more mundane aspects of their chosen

profession. Their passions for collecting historical books went beyond the physical

attraction of an historical text, although that symbolism cannot be separated from

the meaning of the writings and their current implications. Moreover, they were

eager to transmit their knowledge and their precious historical documents to the

next generation of students in their field of interest and beyond.

In some ways, their profiles were reminiscent of Pasteur who arose from a humble

beginning, strove to obtain an advanced education, became a scholar, excelled in

his profession, made a mark in the world that continues to this day, and aided others

in their quest for knowledge. Perhaps this may explain in part the reason why they

desired to obtain a part of Pasteur, that is, of his *Bibliothèque*.

Furthermore, each of these bibliophiles gained fame for their professional achievements. Three of them became renowned medical specialists: Lawrence

Reynolds, a national leader in radiology; Haskell Norman, a leading psychiatrist;

and Truman Blocker, an internationally recognized trauma surgeon, who

revolutionized the medical care of victims of burn injury in many ways. Two of

these individuals, Harry Ransom and Truman Blocker, rose to lead and significantly

develop institutions of higher learning (a state-wide university system and a state

medical school, respectively) peculiarly enough in the same state.

Each of them was interested in the development of their colleagues and students.

This attribute was particularly marked in Ransom and Blocker but was a significant

aspect of the other bibliophiles in this story. All recognized that the torch of

scholarship had to be passed to those who would follow after they were gone. The

libraries would be a focal point for the development of the new generations of

scholars as well as for the continued enlightenment of those with proven expertise.

However, it is also ironic that the intellectually gifted individuals who came to

possess parts of *la Bibliothèque de Louis Pasteur* probably had very little

knowledge of the sciences of microbiology and immunology that Pasteur pioneered.

Ransom and Dibner knew little about biological sciences or medicine. The other

three, Reynolds, Norman, and Blocker, were excellent physicians, but their

expertise in medicine laid elsewhere: radiology, psychiatry, plastic surgery, and

burn trauma, respectively and not microbiology or immunology.

It is also doubtful that any of them fully comprehended the future impact of those sciences upon the practice of medicine other than the development of vaccines that protected against serious infections. It is also doubtful that they knew the full history of Pasteur's life. But that may pertain to many collectors of ancient, historically important books. In that regard, a colleague remarked while visiting the Truman G. Blocker, Jr. History of Medicine Collections, at least you get a chance to hold and read a book that a famous scientist once held and studied or even created. These bibliophiles, or as some would say bibliomaniacs, were drawn to the symbol of Pasteur, as many historians, physicians, scientists, and other members of the society are today.

But there is a more palpable reason. Scholars in the history of medicine will have an opportunity to examine original works by Pasteur and his colleagues that are located in several institutions.

Chapter 11. Epilogue - Unanswered Questions

"People stop thinking when they cease to read." ~ Denis Diderot

Several important questions concerning *la Bibliothèque de Louis Pasteur* remain to be explored. One of them is whether there were precedents for the relocation of the library of the famous Frenchman from France to another other land.

Relocations of Libraries of Two Other Famous People

There are at least two other precedents. The libraries of the famous and controversial philosopher-historian, critic of organized religions, and humanitarian Voltaire (François-Marie Aroeut) and the philosopher, scientist, humanitarian, and encyclopedist Denis Diderot were purchased by the Empress of Russia, Catherine the Great. After Voltaire's death in 1778, Catherine purchased his library of over six thousand volumes from Voltaire's widowed niece and lover, Madame Denis, for 135,000 pounds. The Empress Catherine purchased Dennis Diderot's library for 16,000 pounds while Diderot was still alive, but she insisted that the library remain with him until his death.

It is of considerable interest that no effort was made by the French Royalty or other wealthy citizens of France to purchase those important collections. Perhaps that was because of the controversies that Voltaire and Diderot engendered by their writings and public declamations. However, in contrast to the openness of the purchases of those historically important libraries by the Empress of Russia, the purchase of *la Bibliothèque de Louis Pasteur* was so secretive that many of the precise details remain hidden or lost forever.

Fate of Pasteur's Library During World War II

Although many of the mysteries concerning *la Bibliothèque de Louis Pasteur* have been resolved, many more questions linger on. One of the main ones concerning the fate of the Library during World War II. How was *la Bibliothèque de Louis Pasteur* protected during World War II when Joseph Louis Pasteur Vallery-Radot was working in the French Resistance and being hunted by the Gestapo? Where was the Library stored and who looked after it? Since the story would be exciting, one would have thought that this tale would have been told shortly after the end of World War II. Indeed, it would have been of great interest to the citizens of France, as well as many others in other countries who greatly admired Pasteur and might have been made into a movie if the content was as full of intrigue as we imagined.

The Sale of Pasteur's Library

And then there was the sale of *la Bibliothèque de Louis Pasteur*. Why was *la Bibliothèque* sold? How were the sales conducted? Was the counsel of important microbiologists or immunologists sought during that crucial time?

At first consideration, it would seem incongruous that *la Bibliothèque de Louis Pasteur* would be permitted to leave France. Apparently, when segments of *la*

Bibliothèque de Louis Pasteur were sold, there was no public disclosure of the intent to sell or of the sales. One could imagine the uproar that would have happened if it were disclosed that *la Bibliothèque de Louis Pasteur* was being dismembered and that significant parts of it were to be sent to distant countries. How wrenching that would have been since Pasteur was a national hero in France at the time and remains so to this day. Surely if an announcement would have been made to place any segment of *la Bibliothèque de Louis Pasteur* for sale, the matter would have caused an uproar not only in France but also in many other Western European countries and in the United States. If that had been the case, it was very likely that a serious attempt would have been made by national and private groups in France to keep *la Bibliothèque de Louis Pasteur* either at *l'Institut Pasteur en Paris*, *l'Bibliothèque nationale de France* or some other national repository in France. However, despite numerous efforts, the individuals who might have shed further light on these issues never knew or could not remember what happened.

But before further examining those questions, it is indicated to review the general state of affairs in France during the decades when plans were made to sell the Library and the period when segments of the Library were sold to the American bibliophiles. The breakup and dispersal of *la Bibliothèque de Louis Pasteur* occurred during a period of great change in France. The overwhelming election of General Charles de Gaulle as the President of France inaugurated a new set of internal and international policies in the nascent Fifth Republic. A new French franc was printed. Many new economic measures were instituted. Many workers from French colonies in Africa came to work in France. They comprised about eight percent of the total population. The economy boomed for some years. France developed an atomic bomb and invested a great deal in the development of nuclear energy plants to provide energy for the country.

President de Gaulle pushed for a confederation of European States that excluded the influence of the United States, Great Britain, and the Soviet Union. His vision was to restore the past glories of the great European empires by creating a confederation of all European nations. His stance was summarized in a speech that he delivered in Strasbourg in 1959.

"Oui, c'est l'Europe, depuis l'Atlantique jusqu'à l'Oural, c'est toute l'Europe, qui décidera du destin du monde." (*"Yes, it is Europe, from the Atlantic to the Urals, it is Europe, it is the whole of Europe, that will decide the destiny of the world."*)

However, that vision may have been somewhat blurred by the civil war in Algeria that drew a great deal of international criticism. In that regard, Algerian rebel paratroopers threatened an invasion of France in 1961, and President Charles de Gaulle was the target of several assassination attempts, one of which nearly succeeded. After Algeria became independent in July 1962, an amnesty was issued covering all crimes committed during the war, including the use of torture. Subsequently, some 900,000 French settlers and Algerians who fought for France left Algeria to resettle in France.

During the latter part of the 1960s, the economy of France improved a great deal. That air of optimism over the economy however was being replaced in the 1970s by the realization that France was no longer one of the powerful countries because of the continued ascendancy of the United States in international affairs, science, and to a great extent in modern culture. That was worsened by the policies of the French Government that weakened the European Union and the relationships with the United States and Great Britain. The situation was further confused because of the Cold War, as both the Soviet Union and the West knew that France sought a position that was between socialism and capitalism.

Furthermore, Germany rose from the ashes of the Second World War to become the dominant industrial power in Europe. In contrast, the centuries old idea of French dominance in the world was eroding as they lost their foreign colonies. Also, France fell behind in science and technology. Whereas the French language was one of the dominant forms of speech and writing for centuries, in the last half of the twentieth century, English became the *lingua franca* in Western societies and beyond. The French understandably feared that their language was becoming imperiled because of the introduction of many English terms in science, the technologies, and the general culture. Their efforts to defend their language in a sense further separated them from the main stream of western culture.

All of these events were occurring in France when *la Bibliothèque de Louis Pasteur* was in the process of being dispersed to the United States. Furthermore, during that period, there were vigorous debates in the public media concerning many contentious

issues such as reformation of the penal system, feminism, the failure of many recent

immigrants to adapt to the "French Culture," and the plight of psychiatric patients.

The association with those momentous events suggests that leaders in the French

Government and most enlightened citizens in the country were too preoccupied with

those many matters to consider the fate of the library of one of the most famous

Frenchmen of all times.

Joseph Louis Pasteur Vallery-Radot's Role

But in finality, the fate of *la Bibliothèque de Louis Pasteur* was in the hands of his

sole remaining descendant, his grandson, Joseph Louis Pasteur Vallery-Radot. In

retrospect, the most straightforward course would have been to give the priceless

collection to the famous institute that Pasteur founded in the late nineteenth century.

Surely, the leaders of the Pasteur Institute would have been thrilled to receive the

precious documents. Undoubtedly, Vallery-Radot, his wife, the members of the

Institute, the officers and other members of the French Academy of Science, other

key scientists, and many members of the French Government would have assembled

at *l'Institut Pasteur en Paris* to commemorate the occasion. The life and

accomplishments of Pasteur would have been praised by leading French

microbiologists and immunologists of the day and by medical historians. The story

of Pasteur's grandson including his life as a physician scientist, his heroic service to

the French Resistance during the German occupation of France in the Second World

War, and his service in the French Government after that war ended would have been told in glowing detail. Undoubtedly, it would also have been revealed in that story how Vallery-Radot protected his grandfather's precious library while the infamous Gestapo hunted him during the five-year German occupation.

And if for some reason, *l'Institut Pasteur en Paris* would have been unable to receive *la Bibliothèque de Louis Pasteur*, then the collection could have been temporarily or permanently housed in *l'Bibliothèque nationale de France*, particularly since Pasteur's laboratory notebooks were given to *l'Bibliothèque*. But neither possibility came to pass.

It was extraordinary that Vallery-Radot never discussed a possible sale of the library of his esteemed grandfather in public, and if he did so in private, that part of the story never emerged. Furthermore, from scraps of correspondence from Parisian book dealers and a few other pieces of information that were uncovered, the entire matter of the sale of *la Bibliothèque de Louis Pasteur* was suppressed for many decades later. In fact, even the curators of the Library at *l'Institut Pasteur en Paris* were unaware of the dispersal of *la Bibliothèque de Louis Pasteur* until recently.

And finally, there was the death of Vallery-Radot that occurred shortly before the sale of the library of his famous grandfather. Was Vallery-Radot too ill from his cardiovascular disease to prepare the final disposition of *la Bibliothèque de Louis Pasteur*? Was his wife too distressed or otherwise unprepared to help make the decision? That we may never know.

Another related reason why Vallery-Radot or his wife may have decided to relinquish control of his grandfather's library was because of financial difficulties. Although the French economy improved dramatically after the Second World War, Vallery-Radot's financial situation during that period was unclear, particularly since he was principally involved in leading a public health initiative for the county and was helping to rejuvenate his grandfather's institute. It may be germane that Vallery-Radot died in 1970, whereas his wife Jacqueline lived for 16 more years. If he realized that his wife might survive for at least several years after his death, he may have decided to sell his grandfather's library in order to provide enough funds for her needs.

Some evidence indicates that segments of *la Bibliothèque de Louis Pasteur* were sold at separate times. But if that occurred, the exact dates concerning most of the transactions, the costs, and possible stipulations concerning who should be allowed to purchase some or all of the library remain shrouded in mystery. That is because some of the book dealers maintained no records, whereas the other book dealers no longer exist. A closely related question is how it was decided to divide *la Bibliothèque de Louis Pasteur* or whether that came about by chance.

Apparently, there were no public announcements from the book dealers that the Library would be sold. Instead, as was the habit of that day, bibliophiles who had purchased historical documents in the past, the likes of Dibner, Reynolds, Blocker, Norman, and Ransom, were told of the upcoming sales of parts of *la Bibliothèque*.

The details of the transactions of sale of the several segments of *la Bibliothèque de Louis Pasteur*, and the conditions of the sales to the bookstores and to the eventual owners of these priceless documents remain unclear. What, if any, were the stipulations placed on the bookstores as to the types of clients who might purchase the separate parts of *la Bibliothèque de Louis Pasteur*? How would each part of *la Bibliothèque de Louis Pasteur* be maintained or made available to future Pasteur scholars? Answers to all of these questions are important to the final unraveling of the mystery of *la Bibliothèque de Louis Pasteur*.

Did The Bibliophiles Ever Meet?

Since Bern Dibner, Harry Ransom, Haskell Norman, Lawrence Reynolds, and Truman Blocker lived at the same times and were keenly interested in the history of medicine in general and went to great lengths to obtain parts of *la Bibliothèque de Louis Pasteur*, the question arose whether they had an opportunity to meet each other and discuss their mutual interests. Bern Dibner and Lawrence Reynolds most likely were unaware of the other bibliophiles who were part of this story. In contrast, Haskell Norman and Truman Blocker were aware of each other since Haskell Norman's son, Jeremy, was the book dealer who sold the part of *la Bibliothèque de Louis Pasteur* that eventually came to the University of Texas Medical Branch at Galveston. As previously indicated, Truman Blocker knew that Haskell Norman had originally purchased the collection and then willed it to his son Jeremy. In addition, their interests crossed in another important way since the University of Texas

Medical Branch Library obtained a very important, extensive collection of historical documents concerning psychiatry that were originally owned by Haskell Norman. However, there is no evidence that Haskell Norman and Truman Blocker ever met, even though Blocker had visited San Francisco where Haskell and Jeremy Norman lived.

Harry Ransom and Truman Blocker knew each other quite well since Ransom was the Chancellor of the University of Texas System at the same time that Blocker was the President of the University of Texas Medical Branch during the late 1960s and early 1970s. Each of them knew that they shared a common mania for historical materials. However, Truman Blocker was unaware that Harry Ransom independently obtained an important part of *la Bibliothèque de Louis Pasteur*. By the time that Blocker obtained the part that currently resides in the University of Texas Medical Branch, Ransom had already passed away. Why Blocker was unaware of what Ransom had obtained is another unanswered question concerning the mystery.

Analysis of La Bibliothèque de Louis Pasteur Yet to Come

If it is assumed that most of *la Bibliothèque de Louis Pasteur* has been "reassembled", then there are new opportunities for historians and physicians to more thoroughly investigate this aspect of Pasteur. For example, it should be informative to study the annotations that Pasteur made in books, journal articles (Figure 26), or letters in his library. But then the question remains: what is missing?

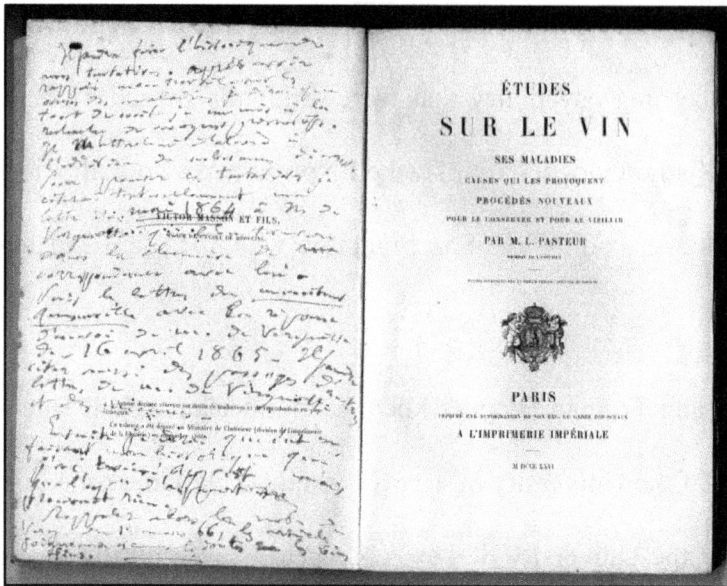

Figure 28. A reprint of Pasteur's article concerning his study of the cause of fermentation of wine. The page before the article contains Pasteur's comments.

Are Parts of Pasteur's Library Still Missing?

Another important question is whether other parts of *la Bibliothèque de Louis Pasteur* are still missing. It is strange that major parts of *la Bibliothèque de Louis Pasteur* were dispersed to California, Texas, and Alabama and that each of these important libraries contains valuable documents, whereas no parts of *la Bibliothèque de Louis Pasteur* went to more well-established institutions such as those located in London, New York, or Boston. It would therefore not be surprising that some other parts of this famous library may yet emerge in hitherto unsuspected places that may be in the United States or elsewhere. In that respect, if other parts of *la Bibliothèque de Louis Pasteur* are housed in sites other than the known ones, perhaps that information will surface because of the study of this book. Then the information could be disseminated to all who are interested in Pasteur, his works, his Library, and the origins of the sciences of microbiology and immunology.

Final Words

It has been a privilege to investigate this fascinating, historically important subject. To do so, it was necessary learn more about not only Pasteur and his descendants but also about many aspects of about the history of France during the Second World War and in the two decades thereafter, the book dealers who dealt with the sale of *la Bibliothèque de Louis Pasteur*, the lives and accomplishments of the bibliophiles who purchased the segments of the Library, and the contents of the entire Library. As the book was being assembled, it began to take on a life of its own. Indeed, the final product seemed to exceed the sum of its parts.

Explorations of the historical documents of famous people in a sense are becoming less possible in the digital age in which we live. Most letters are no longer written by hand. Typewriters have nearly disappeared. If correspondence is carried out, it is most often performed by emails or via other digital devices. Records of such correspondence are maintained for variable lengths of time in computers, but unless that the documents are stored safely elsewhere, they may be lost when the computer is gone. Thus, the elements of personal contacts may disappear quickly.

An exploration of the dispersal of the library of one of the most famous scientists of all times are comparatively rare. No one dreamed that such a book would have been contemplated until this century. As our accidental explorations began, the complexity of the story was discovered. It is complex because of the fascinating people in medicine and the humanities who were involved and how their lives were almost as illuminating as Pasteur's. Hopefully the readers will also find it so and that some may, in time, be able to add to the story of the mystery of *la Bibliothèque de Louis Pasteur*.

Perhaps the following will help to sum up what we have learned and are yet to learn about Louis Pasteur and his library.

Pasteur, innovator of microbiology and immunology, was a mystery in many ways,

For before he became a scientist, he came from a poor family in his early days.

And how he came to rise to fame,

Is a mystery that still remains.

We thought that a study of his library would provide a clue,

But that would mean going to Paris by crossing the ocean blue.

And we were not alone, until a famous surgeon asked that I reconceive.

The "General" asked in a whimsical way, "Armond where is Pasteur's Library?"

I saluted him -mentally that is - and with more than it took for a glance,

I responded with a little chuckle – why of course it's in France.

And the General laughed, as was his style,

When he wished to make a point worthwhile.

And told me where in the USA that a portion was,

And how if it was brought to Galveston that would be first class.

But the complete answer to the Pasteur Library question,

Took many a moon and much reflection.

For the puzzle concerning Pasteur's Library went unsolved for a long time,

Since puzzle pieces were hard to find, and our ideas were not sublime.

But then the bibliophiles with their parts of Pasteur's Library were found,

And how they brought them to America and their stories were quite profound.

But why the Library was sold was not completely revealed,

And how was it protected during World War II by Pasteur's sole remaining kin?

That was a story that we could not hope to know, much to our chagrin.

But perhaps someone who has the knowledge and reads this tome,

Will bring some answers to this puzzle home.

And then hopefully more will be enlightened,

The puzzle might be resolved, and our understanding heightened.

References

1. Oertling SB, Marlin RO IV, Goldman AS. The mysterious fate of *La Bibliothèque de Louis* Pasteur. J Med Biography 2014; 22:195-204.

2. Kapr A. Johannes Gutenberg: The Man and His Invention. Leicester: Scolar Press, 1996.

3. Priestley J. An Account of Further Discoveries in Air. Philosophical Transactions 1775; 65:384–94.

4. Lavoisier A. Traité élémentaire de Chimie, Présenté dans un ordre nouveau, et d'Aprês Découvertes Modernes. Paris: Cuchet Libraire, 1789.

5. Hahn R. Pierre Simon Laplace, 1749-1827: A Determined Scientist. Boston: Harvard University Press, 2005.

6. Schmalstieg FC Jr, Goldman AS. Metchnikoff and Ehrlich: The Centennial of the 1908 Nobel Prize in Physiology or Medicine. J Med Biogr 2008; 16:96-103.

7. Schmalsteig FC, Goldman AS. Jules Bordet. A bridge to the twentieth century. J Med Biogr 2009; 17:217-24.

8. Bibel DJ, Chen TH. Diagnosis of plaque: an analysis of the Yersin-Kitasato controversy. Bacteriolo Rev 1976; 40:633–51.

9. Simond M, Godley ML, Mouriquand PDE. Paul-Louis Simond and his discovery of plague transmission by rat fleas: A centenary. J Roy Soc Med

1998; 91:101-4.

10.   Hawgood BJ. Albert Calmette (1863-1933) and Camille Guérin (1872-1961):
      The C and G of BCG vaccine. J Med Biogr 2007; 15:139-46.

11.   Nye ER. Alphonse Laveran (1845–1922): discoverer of the malarial parasite
      and Nobel laureate, 1907. J Med Biogr 2002; 10:81-7.

12.   Summers WC. Bacteriophage research: early history. In: Kutter E, Sulakvelidze
      A, eds. Bacteriophages: Biology and Applications. Eds. Boca Raton, Florida:
      CRC Press, 2004.

13.   Lwoff AM. Les Bactéries Lysogènes et la Notion de Provirus. Paris: Masson,
      1954.

14.   Barré-Sinoussi F, Chermann JC, Rey F, Nugeyre MT, Chamaret S, Gruest J,
      Dauguet C, Axler-Blin C, Vézinet-Brun F, Rouzioux C, Rozenbaum W,
      Montagnier L. Isolation of a T-lymphotropic retrovirus from a patient at risk
      for acquired immune deficiency syndrome (AIDS). Science 1983; 220:868–71.

15.   Landsteiner K, Levaditi C. La transmission de la paralysie infantile aux singes.
      Comptes Rendus des Seances de la Societe de Biologie et de ses Filiales 1909;
      67:592-4.

16.   Scharnhorst G. Horatio Alger, Jr. Woodbridge, Conn: Twayne Publishers,
      1980.

17.   Debré P (Translated from French into English by Forster E). Louis Pasteur.

Baltimore MD: Johns Hopkins University Press, 1998.

18. Schmalstieg FC, Goldman AS. The birth of the science of immunology. J Med Biogr 2010; 18:88-98.

19. Laurent, Auguste (or Augustin).Complete Dictionary of Scientific Biography. 2008. Encyclopedia.com. 4 Sep. 2013 <http://www.encyclopedia.com>.

20. Chastain BB. Jean-Baptiste-André Dumas. French Chemist. Encyclopaedia Britannica, 2013.

21. Crosland MP. Biot, Jean-Baptiste. Dictionary of Scientific Biography 2. New York: Charles Scribner's Sons. 1970–80, pages 133-140.

22. Charlot, Colette; Flahaut Jean. Antoine Jérôme Balard. The man. Revue d'histoire de la pharmacie 2003; 51:251-64.

23. Pasteur L. Transformation des acides tartriques en acide racémique. Paris: Imprimerie de Mallet-Bachelier, 1853.

24. Pasteur, L. Mémoire sur les acides aspartique et malique. Paris: Imprimerie de Bachelier, 1852.

25. Pasteur L. Recherches sur la dissymétrie moléculaire des produits organiques naturels. Paris: Imprimerie de Ch. Lahure et Cie, 1860.

26. Geison GI. *The Private Science of Louis Pasteur*. Princeton, New Jersey: Princeton University Press, 1995.

27. Aristotle. History of Animals, Book V, Part 1, circa 350 BCE.

28. Harvey W. Exercitationes de Generatione Animalium. London: Typis Du–Gardianis, Impensis Octaviani Pulleyn, 1651.

29. Lopata A. History of the egg in embryology. J Mammalian Ova Res 2009; 26:2-9.

30. Holmyard, EJ. Makers of Chemistry. Oxford: Oxford University Press, 1931.

31. Nutton V. The reception of Fracastoro's theory of contagion: The seed that fell among thorns? Osiris 1990; 6:196–234.

32. Redi F. *Experienza Intorno all Generazione degl'Insetto.* Translated from the Italian Edition by Mab Bigelow. Chicago: The Open Court Publishing Company, 1909.

33. Dobell C. Antony van Leeuwenhoek and His 'Little Animals. New York: Russell & Russell, Inc., 1958.

34. Raynaud D. La correspondence de F-A Pouchet avec les membres de l'Académie des Sciences: une réévaluation du débat sur la génération spontanée. European J Sociology 1999; 40:257-76.

35. Springer A. The microorganisms of the soil. Nature 1892; 46:576–9.

36. Darwin C. On the Origin of Species by Means of Natural Selection or The Preservation of Favoured Races in the Struggle for Life. London: John Murray, Albemarle Street, 1859.

37. Pasteur L. Corpuscules organisesqui existant dans l'atmosphere, examen de la doctrine des generations spontanées. Extrait des Annales de Chimie et de Physique 1862; 64:5-110.

38. Pasteur L. Études sur le vin, ses maladies, causes qui les provoquent, procédés nouveaux pour le conserver et pour le vieillir. Paris: Imprimerie impériale, 1866.

39. Brock WH. Justus von Liebig: The Chemical Gatekeeper. Cambridge: Cambridge University Press, 2002.

40. Pasteur L. Études sur la maladies des vers a soie. Paris: Gauthier-Villars, Imprimeur-Libraire de Bureau des Longitudes, 1870.

41. Pasteur L. Sur les maladies virulentes, el en particulier sur la maladie appelee vulgairement cholera des poules. Comptes Rendus Herdomaires des Séances de l'Academie des Sciences 1880; 19:239-48.

42. Pasteur L. Sur la vaccination Charbonneuse. Comptes rendus des séances del l' Academie des Sciences 1882; 92:1-8.

43. Pasteur L. Résultats de l'application de la methode pour prévenir la rage, après morsure. Comptes redus de l'Academie des Sciences 1886; 55:1-3

44. Rocchietta S. Casimir-Joseph Davaine (1812-1882), pioniere della microbiologia medica. Minerva Medicine 1970; 61:11.

45. Toussaint H, De l'immunité pour le charbon, acquise à la suite d'inoculations

préventives. Comptes rendus de l'Académie des sciences 1880; 91:135-7.

46.   Carter KD. Koch's postulates in relation to the work of Jacob Henle and Edwin Klebs. Medical History 1985; 29:533-74.

47.   Koch R. Die Aetiologie der Milzbrand-Krankheit, begründet auf die Entwicklungsgeschichte des Bacillus Anthracis. Beiträge zur Biologie der Pflanzen 1876; 2:277-310.

48.   Koch R. Die Aetiologie der Tuberculose. Berliner klinische Wochenschrift 1882; 19:221-30.

49.   Pasteur L De l'attenuation des virus. Quatrième Congrès Internationale de l' Hygiène et Démographie. Geneve 1882; 1:127-49.

50.   Koch R. Über die Milzbrandimpfung. Eine Entgegnung auf den von Pasteur in Genf gehaltenen Vortrag. Gesammelte Werke 1882; 1:207-31.

51.   Howard M. The Franco–Prussian War: The German Invasion of France 1870–1871. New York: Routledge, 1991. sci tech Off int Epiz 1994; 13:361-727.

52.   Wasik B, Murphy M. Rabid: A Cultural History of the World's Most Diabolical Virus. London: Penguin Books, 2013.

53.   Dietzschold B, Li J, Faber M, Schnell M. Concepts in the pathogenesis of rabies. Future Virol 2008; 3: 481–90.

54.   Serendipity and the Three Princes from the Peregrinaggio of 1557. Edited, with an Introduction and Notes, by Theodore G. Remer. Preface by W. S. Lewis.

Norman OK: University of Oklahoma Press, 1965.

55. Hebraic Literature: Translations from the Talmud, Midrashim, and Kabbala, chapter II.

56. Crump JA. Salmonella Infections (Including Typhoid Fever). In: Goldman's Cecil Medicine. Ed, Goldman L, Schafer AI. 24th Edition. Philadelphia: Saunders Elsevier, 2008.

57. Cohn DV. Pasteur. Louisville: University of Louisville, 2004.

58. Howard M. The Franco–Prussian War: The German Invasion of France 1870–1871. New York: Routledge, 1991.

59. Osler W. The Evolution of Modern Medicine. A Series of Lectures delivered at Yale University on the Stillman Foundation, April 1913. In: Vallery-Radot R. Louis Pasteur - His Life and Labours. D. New York: Doubleday, 1914.

60. Goldman D. Our Genes. Our Choices. How Genotype and Gene Interactions Affect Behavior. Waltham, Mass: Academic Press, 2012.

61. Louis Pasteur Vallery-Radot. http://www.academie-francaise.fr/les-immortels/louis-pasteur-vallery-radot?fauteuil=24&election=12-10-1944

62. Vallery-Radot P, Wolfromin R, Charpin I, Halpern BN. Maladies Allergiques. Paris, France: Flammarion Medicine, 1963.

63. Green R. Vive la France: The French Resistance During World War II. New York: F Watts, 1995.

64. Kelly MH. The Cultural and Intellectual Rebuilding of France after the Second World War. Basingstoke, UK: Palgrave Macmillan, 2004.

65. D. Zallen, the Rockefeller Foundation and French Research, Cahiers pour l'histoire du CNRS, 1989-5.

    http://www.vjf.cnrs.fr/histcnrs/pdf/cahiers-cnrs/zallen.pdf.

66. Gimbel J. The Origins of the Marshall Plan. Palo Alto, CA: Stanford University Press, 1976.

67. Stephens HW. The Texas City Disaster, 1947. Austin, Texas: The University of Texas Press, 1997.

68. Blocker V, Blocker TG Jr, The Texas City Disaster: A survey of 3,000 casualties. Am J Surgery 1949; 78:756-71.

69. Garfield E. To remember Chauncey D. Leake. Essays of an Information Scientist Philadelphia PA: ISI Press1978; 411-21.

70. Norman HF. My Education as a Bibliophile. Jeremy Norman's History of Science, Medicine and Technology. 19 Jan. 2011 www.historyofscience.com

71. Norman HF. One Hundred Books Famous in Medicine. Edited by Hope Mayo. New York: The Grolier Club, 1995.

72. Metchnikoff E. Immunity in Infectious Dis*eases*. Cambridge: Cambridge University Press, 1905.

73. Donné A. Cours de Microscopie. Vol I et Atlas No. I, Paris: Bailliére, 1844-

1845.

74. Darwin C, Wallace AR. On the tendency of species to form varieties; and on the perpetuation of varieties and species by natural means of selection. Journal of the Proceedings of the Linnean Society of London. Zoology 1858; 3:45–62.

75. Schmalstieg FC, Goldman AS. The birth of the science of immunology. J Med Biogr 2010; 18:88-98.

76. Cohen IB. Award of the 1976 Sarton Medal to Bern Dibner, ISIS; 1977: 68.

77. Petroski H. From connections to collections. Am Scientist 1998; 86416-20.

78. Holton G, Eloges SSS. Bern Dibner, 1878-1978. ISIS; 1988; 79: 298.

79. Hawes LE. Bern Dibner—Twentieth Century Humanist. Octavo 1973; No. 4.

80. Friedlander GD. The Burndy Library: window on the history of science. IEEE Spectrum, March 1970.

81. Huntington Library Website and Personal communication with Dr. Daniel Lewis, Chief Curator of Manuscripts (Science, Medicine and Technology) Philip Weimerskirsch, former Assistant Director of the Burndy Library, and Brent Dibner, grandson of Bern and Billie Dibner.

82. Pasteur: Exemplaires Personnels de ses Ouvrages relies pour lui et Enriches de Manuscrits Autographes. Son Microscope. Photographies Originales, Alain Brieux Catalogue, between 1970-1986; personal communication from Catherine Wehrey, Huntington Library, Dibner Reader Services Assistant.

83. Personal communication from Philip Weimerskirsch, former Assistant Director of the Burndy Library.

84. Weaver B, Butt MC. Dr. Lawrence Reynolds and his medical history collection. Ala J Med Sciences 1984; 21:311-447.

85. Schuman H. A dream come true: The Lawrence Reynolds Collection. B Med Libr Assoc 1959; 47:235-252.

86. Gribben A. Harry Huntt Ransom. An Intellect in Motion. Austin, Texas: The University of Texas Press, 2008.

87. Hobson A. Great Libraries. New York: GP Putnam's Sons, 1970.

88. Wood J. Personal History. Shelf life. Packing up my father-in-law's library. New Yorker 2011, November 7.

89. Mendel GJ. Versuche über Pflanzenhybriden. Brünn: Naturforschenden Verein Brünn 1866.

90. Henig RM. The Monk in the Garden: The Lost and Found Genius of Gregor Mendel, the Father of Modern Genetics. Boston: Houghton Mifflin Harcourt, 2009.

91. Darwin C. The Variation of Animals and Plants Under Domestication. London: John Murray, 1868.

146

Appendix A - Locations of *la Bibliothèque de Louis Pasteur*

l'Musée Pasteur a l'Institut Pasteur en Paris
Physical Address: 25 rue du Docteur Roux, 75015 Paris, France

Telephone Number: +33 (0) 1 45 68 82 83

Email Address: musee@pasteur.fr

Website: www.pasteur.fr/en/institut-pasteur/pasteur-museum

l'Bibliotheque Nationale de France
Physical Address: Quai François Mauriac, 75013 Paris, France

Telephone Number: +33 (0) 1 53 79 55 00

Email Address: accueil@bnf.fr

Website: www.bnf.fr

Huntington Library in San Mateo, California
Physical Address: 1151 Oxford Road San Marino, CA 91108

Telephone Number: (626) 405-2100

Email Address: reference@huntington.org

Website: www.huntington.org

Harry Ransom Center, University of Texas
Physical Address: 300 West 21st Street, Austin, Texas

Mailing Address: 300 West 21st Street, P.O. Drawer 7219, Austin, Texas 78713-7219

Telephone Number: (512) 471-8944

Fax Number: (512) 471-9646

Email Address: webmail@hrc.utexas.edu

Website: www.hrc.utexas.edu

Reynolds-Finley Historical Library, University of Alabama in Birmingham

Physical Address: 1700 University Boulevard, Birmingham, Alabama

Mailing Address: 1720 2nd Avenue South, Birmingham, Alabama 35294-0013

Telephone Number: (205) 934-4475

Fax Number: (205) 975-8476

Website: www.uab.edu/reynolds

The Truman G Blocker, Jr. History of Medicine Collections, Moody Medical Library, University of Texas Medical Branch at Galveston.

Physical Address: 914 Market Street, Galveston, Texas

Mailing Address: 301 University Boulevard, Galveston, Texas 77555-1035

Telephone Number: (409) 772-2397

Fax Number: (409) 765-9852

Email Address: askus@utmb.libanswers.com

Website: www.utmb.edu/ar/Blocker History of Medicine

Appendix B – Materials Held by Selected Libraries

The Truman G Blocker, Jr. History of Medicine Collections, Moody Medical Library, University of Texas Medical Branch at Galveston.
Included in the purchase of this collection are items that were published after Pasteur's death, relating to immunology and microbiology.

Some items from this collection have been digitized with Federal funds from the National Library of Medicine, National Institutes of Health, under Contract No. HHSN-276-2011-00007-C with the Houston Academy of Medicine-Texas Medical Center Library. www.utmb.edu/ar/Blocker History of Medicine/Digital/Pasteur

1. Addison, T., & University of Edinburgh. (1815). *Dissertatio medica inauguralis quaedam de syphilide et hydrargyro complectens: Quam ... ex auctoritate ... D. Georgii Baird ... pro gradu doctoris.* Edinburgi: Abernethy & Walker.

2. British Medical Association. (1910). *The Evolution of Antiseptic Surgery: An historical sketch of the use of antiseptics from the earliest times.* London: Burroughs Wellcome and Co.

3. Arneth, J. (1904). *Die neutrophilen weissen Blutkörperchen bei Infektions-Krankheiten.* Jena: Fischer.

4. Arrhenius, Prof. Dr. Svante. (1889). *Anwendungen der physikalischen Chemie in der Immunitatslehre.*

5. Astruc, J. (1761). *Traité des maladies des femmes: Où l'on a tâché de joindre à une théorie solide la pratique la plus sûre & la mieux éprouvée.* A Paris: Chez P. Guillaume Cavelier, libraire. (6 volumes)

6. Astruc, J. (1736). *De morbis venereis libri sex: In quibus disseritur tum de origine, propagatione & contagione horumce affectuum in genere: tum de singulorum natura, aetiologia & therapeia, cum brevi analysi & epicrisi operum plerorumque quae de eodem argumento scripta sunt.* Lutetiae Parisiorum: Apud Guillelmum Cavelier.

7. Bary, A. (1885). *Vorlesungen über Bacterien.* Leipzig: Engelmann.

8. Bassi, A. (1837). *Del mal del segno calcinaccio o moscardino, malattia che affligge i bachi da seta e sul modo di liberarne le bigattaje anche le più ifestate.* Milano: P.A. Molina.

9. Rumsey, J. (1827). *Some account of the life and character of the late Thomas Bateman, M.D., F.L.S: Physician to the Public Dispensary, and to the Fever Institution in London.* London: Printed for Longman, Rees, Orme, Brown, and Green.

10. Hosack, D., & Francis, J. W. (1810). *The American medical and philosophical register: Or, Annals of medicine, natural history, agriculture and the arts.* New York: E. Sargeant. (4 volumes)

11. Beddoes, T., Biggs, B., Ewart, J., Lavoisier, A. L., Thornton, R. J., & Withering, W. (1794). Letters from Dr. Withering ... Dr. Ewart ... Dr. Thornton ... and Dr. Biggs: ... together with some other papers, supplementary to two publications on asthma, consumption, fever, and other diseases. Bristol: Bulgin and Rosser [etc.

12. Bell, B., & Campbell, R. (1795). A treatise on gonorrhoea virulenta, and lues venerea. Philadelphia: Printed for Robert Campbell, bookseller.

13. Besredka, A. (1927). Local Immunization; Specific Dressings. Baltimore: Williams & Wilkins Company.

14. Pettenkofer, M. & Stanton A. Friedberg, M.D. Rare Book Collection of Rush University Medical Center at the University of Chicago. (1855). Untersuchungen und Beobachtungen über die Verbreitungsart der Cholera nebst Betrachtungen über Massregeln: Derselben Einhalt zu thun. München: Cotta.

15. Bier, A. (1903). Hyperämie als Heilmittel. Leipzig: F.C.W. Vogel.

16. Great Britain. (1805). First [-second] report of the Board of Health: An outline of a plan to prevent the spreading of the plague, or other contagious diseases. London: s.n.

17. Rosenthal, J and Senator, H. (1877). Centralblatt fur die medicinischen Wissenchaften. Berlin: Verlag von August Hirschwald.

18. Bordeu, T., Bordeu, A., & Bordeu, F. (1775). Recherches sur les maladies chroniques: Leurs rapports avec les maladies aiguës, leurs périodes, leur nature: & sur la maniere dont on les traite aux eaux minérales de Bareges, & des autres sources de l'Aquitaine. Paris: Ruault.

19. Bretonneau, P. F. (1826). Des inflammations spéciales du tissu muqueux: Et en particulier de la diphthérite, ou inflammation pelliculaire, connue sous le nom de croup, d'angine maligne, d'angine gangréneuse, etc. Paris: Crevot.

20. Bright, R. (1813). De erysipelate contagioso. Edinburgi: Excudebat R. Allan.

21. Bruce, J. M. (1913). The Harveian oration on the influence of Harvey's work in the development of the doctrine of infection and immunity: Delivered before the Royal College of Physicians of London, on October 18, 1913. London: Cassell.

22. Buist, J. B. (1886). The life history of the micro-organisms associated with variola and vaccinia. Edinburgh: printed by Neill and Company

23. Bulloch, William ed. (1906). Studies in Pathology: Written by alumni to celebrate the quarter-centenary of the University of Aberdeen and the quarter-centenary of the chair of pathology therein. Aberdeen.

24. Burgess, A. H. (1941). Development of provincial medical education illustrated in the life and work of Charles White of Manchester. London. (Hunterian Oration)

25. Bernard, N., & Nègre, L. (1939). Albert Calmette: Sa vie, son oeuvre scientifique. Paris: Masson.

26. Campbell, Anna Montgomery (1931). The black death and men of learning. New York: Columbia University Press.

27. Carey, M. (1794). A short account of the malignant fever: Lately prevalent in Philadelphia. Philadelphia: Printed by the author.

28. Carroll, J. (1903). Remarks on the history, cause, and mode of transmission of yellow fever and the occurrence of similar types of fatal fevers in places where yellow fever is not known to have existed. Carlisle, Pa: Association of Military Surgeons.

29. Reed, W., Carroll, J., & American Public Health Association. (1903). The etiology of yellow fever, an addendum, [Pamphlet 7]. Chicago: Press of American Medical Association.

30. Carroll, J., & Daniels, W. B. (1903). The transmission of yellow fever: Read at the Fifty-fourth Annual Session of the American Medical Association, in the Section on Practice of Medicine, and approved for publication by the Executive Committee,

Drs. W.S. Thayer, J.M. Anders and Frank A. Jones. Chicago: American Medical Association Press.

31. Carroll, J. (1905). Yellow fever: A popular lecture. American Journal of Medicine *9(22)*. Philadelphia.

32. Carroll, J. (1905). Lessons to be learned from the present outbreak of yellow fever. Chicago: American Medical Association.

33. Major James Carroll, M.D., U.S.A. Addresses by Drs. H.A. Kelly; W.H. Welch; W.S. Thayer; Surg.-Gen. Sternberg, U.S.A.; H.H. Donnally; A.F.A. King; S. Ruffin; C.E. Munroe; and J.O. Skinner. (1908). Bulletin of the Johns Hopkins Hospital 19(202). Baltimore.

34. Carroll, J. (1902). The treatment of yellow fever: American Medical Association.

35. Catlin, G. (1862). The breath of life, or mal-respiration: And its effects upon the enjoyments & life of man. London: Trübner & Co.

36. Great Britain & Chadwick, E. (1842). Report to Her Majesty's principal Secretary of State for the Home Department. London: Clowes.

37. Charrin, A. (1889). La maladie pyocyanique. Paris: Steinheil.

38. Great Britain. (1850). Report of the General Board of Health on the epidemic cholera of 1848 & 1849. London: W. Clowes.

39. Cohnheim, J. (1877). Vorlesungen über allgemeine Pathologie: Ein Handbuch für Aerzte und Studirende. Berlin: Hirschwald.

40. Cohnheim, J. (1880). Die Tuberkulose vom Standpunkte der Infectionslehre. Leipzig: Edelmann

41. Cohnheim, J. (1867). Ueber Entzündung und Eiterung. Berlin.

42. Cornil, V., & Babeş, V. (1886). Les bactéries et leur role dans l'anatomie et l'histologie pathologiques des maladies infectieuses. Paris: F. Alcan.

43. Craigie, D. (1830). Three cases of ulcerative destruction of the coats of the stomach. Edinburgh Medical and Surgical Journal *125*.

44. Craigie, D. & Royal Infirmary of Edinburgh. (1834). Report of the cases treated during the course of clinical lectures delivered at the Royal Infirmary in the session *1832-1833*. Edinburgh: s.n. (in folder twice as 0055 and 0058)

45. Craigie, D. (1833). Apothecaries' act. Edinburgh.

46. Craigie, D. (1838). *Critical analysis [of] Lecons de clinique medicale faites a l Hotel-Dieu de Paris Par. A.F. Chomel.* Edinburgh.

47. Craigie, D. & Royal Infirmary of Edinburgh. (1836). Report of the cases treated during the course of clinical lectures delivered at the Royal Infirmary in the session 1834-35. Edinburgh: s.n.

48. Craigie, D. & Royal Infirmary of Edinburgh. (1837). Clinical report of the cases treated in the fever ward, no. 9, of the Royal Infirmary, Edinburgh, during the year 1836-1837. Edinburgh: s.n.

49. Craigie, D. (1841). Cases and observations illustrative of the nature of gangrene of the lungs. Edinburgh: J. Stark.

50. Craigie, D. (1843). Notice of a febrile disorder which has prevailed at Edinburgh during the summer of 1843. Edinburgh: s.n.

51. Craigie, D. (1827). Observations, pathological and practical, on whitloe. Edinburgh: s.n.

52. Craigie, D. (1834). Observations, pathological and therapeutic, on a particular species of quinsy or angina. Edinburgh: s.n.

53. Craigie, D. (1832). On the anatomical peculiarities of the sturgeon; (Acipenser Sturio, L.). Edinburgh.

54. Crawfurd, R. H. P. (1914). Plague and pestilence in literature and art. Oxford: Clarendon Press.

55. Crookshank, E. M., & Stanton A. Friedberg, M.D. Rare Book Collection of Rush University Medical Center at the University of Chicago. (1887). Photography of bacteria. New York: J.H. Vail & Co.

56. Currie, J. (1797). Medical reports, on the effects of water, cold and warm, as a remedy in fever, and febrile diseases: Whether applied to the surface of the body, or used as a drink: with observations on the nature of fever; and on the effects of opium, alcohol, and inanition. Liverpool: Printed by J. M'Creery, for Cadell and Davies, London.

57. Currie, W., Palmer, W. T., & College of Physicians of Philadelphia. (1798). Observations on the causes and cure of remitting or bilious fevers: To which is annexed, an abstract of the opinions and practice of different authors; and an appendix, exhibiting facts and reflections relative to the synochus icteroides, or yellow fever. Philadelphia: Printed for the author by William T. Palmer.

58. Dale, H. H. (1935). The Harveian oration on some epochs in medical research: Delivered before the Royal College of Physicians of London on October 18, 1935. London: H.K. Lewis.

59. Darwin, C. Weeks, M., John Murray (Firm)., William Clowes and Sons., Bradbury & Evans., & Edmonds & Remnants. (1859). On the origin of species by means of natural selection, or, The preservation of favoured races in the struggle for life. London: John Murray, Albemarle Street.

60. Davaine, C.-J. (1870). Études sur la genèse et la propagation du charbon. Paris: J.B. Baillière et fils.

61. Davaine, C.-J. (1870). Études sur la contagion du charbon chez les animaux domestiques. Paris: J.B. Baillière et fils.

62. Davaine, C.-J. (1870). De l'incubation des maladies charbonneuses: Et de son rapport avec la quantité de virus inoculé. Paris: J.B. Baillière.

63. Venzmer, G. (1939). Wissenschaft besiegt Mikroben. München: Knorr & Hirth.

64. Hérelle, F. (1921). Le bactériophage; son rôle dans l'immunité. Paris: Masson et cie.

65. Downes, A. and Blunt, T. (1878). On the influence of light upon protoplasm. London: Harrison and sons, printers.

66. Donné, A., & Foucault, L. (1844). Cours de microscopie complémentaire des études médicales, anatomie microscopique et physiologie des fluides de l'économie. Paris: Baillière. (2 volumes).

67. Donné, A. & Foucault, L. (1845). Cours de microscopie complémentaire des études médicales, anatomie microscopique et physiologie des fluides de l'économie: Atlas exécuté d'après nature au microscope-daguerréotype. Paris: J.-B. Baillière.

68. Downes, A., & Blunt, T. P. (1877). Researches on the effect of light upon bacteria and other organisms. London?: s.n.

69. Pasteur, L. (1858). Memoire sur la fermentation appelee lactique. Annales de chimie et de Physique 3(52).

70. Pasteur, L. (1860). Memoire sur la fermentation alcoolique. Paris: Imprimerie de Mallet-Bachelier.

71. Pasteur, L. (1861). Lecons de chimie professees en 1860. Paris: Societe Chimique de Paris.

72. Pasteur, L. (1862). Mémoire sur les corpuscules organizés qui existent dans l'atmosphère, examen de la doctrine des générations spontanées. Annales de Chimie et de Physique 5(64).

73. Pasteur, L. (1870). Études sur la maladie des vers a soie, moyen pratique assure de la combattre et den prévenir le retour. Paris: Gauthier-Villars, Imprimeur-Libraire. (2 volumes)

74. Pasteur, L. and Naumann (1871). Une correspondence entre un savant Français et un savant Prussien pendant la guerre. Paris: Chez les Principaux Libraires.

75. Darwin, C. & Wallace, A. R. (1858). On the tendency of species to form varieties: And on the perpetuation of varieties and species by natural means of selection. London: Linnean Society of London.

76. Pasteur, L., & Bernard, C. (1879). Examen critique d'un écrit posthume de Claude Bernard sur la fermentation. Paris: Gauthier-Villars.

77. Pasteur, L., Faulkner, F., & Robb, D. C. (1879). Studies on fermentation: The diseases of beer, their causes, and the means of preventing them. London: Macmillan & Co.

78. Pasteur, L., & Renan, E. (1882). Discours de réception [à l'Académie française] de M. Louis Pasteur: Réponse de M. Ernest Renen. Paris: C. Lévy.

79. Pasteur, L. & Dumas, J.-B. (1882). Medaille d'honneur offerte à M. Pasteur: Communication de m. le Président de l'Academie des sciences. Paris: Gauthier-Villars.

80. Vallery-Radot, R. (1885). Louis Pasteur; his life and labours. New York: Appleton.

81. Pasteur, L. & Bertrand, J. (1885). Réponse de m. Pasteur ... au discours de m. J. Bertrand: Prononcé ... du jeudi 10 déc. 1885. Paris: typ. Firmin-Didot et cie.

82. Pasteur, L. (1886). Le traitement de la rage. Paris: Marpon et flammarion.

83. Duclaux, E. (1887). Annales de l'institut Pasteur. Paris: G. Masson.

84. Vallery-Radot, R. (1900). La vie de Pasteur. Paris: Hachette et cie.

85. Thomsen, O. & Jensen, V. (1922). Louis Pasteur; Mindeskrift udgivet paa Hundredaarsdagen for hans Fødsel. København: Levin & Munksgaard.

86. Université de Lille. (1923). *Les Travaux de Pasteur: Discours et conferences.* Lille: Marquant.

87. Richet, C. (1923). L'oeuvre de Pasteur. Paris: Alcan.

88. Institut Pasteur (Paris, France). (1939). Institut Pasteur; cinquantenaire de la fondation, 14 Nov. 1888-14 Nov. 1938. Paris (?).

89. Bouley, H.-M. (1882). La nouvelle vaccination: Discours prononcé ... de la Société Nationale d'Acclimatation de France. Paris: Au siège de la Société [impr. Motteroz].

90. Chamberland, C. (1883). Le charbon et la vaccination charbonneuse d'après les travaux récents de M. Pasteur. Paris: B. Tignol. (2 copies)

91. Pasteur, L. (1876). Etudes sur la bière: Ses maladies, causes qui les provoquent, procédé pour la rendre inaltérable; avec une théorie nouvelle de la fermentation. Paris: Gauthier-Villars.

92. Pasteur, L. (1886). Nouvelle communication sur la rage. Paris: G. Masson.

93. Suzor, J. R. (1887). Hydrophobia, an account of M. Pasteur's system: Containing a translation of all his communications on the subject, the technique of his method, and the latest statistical results. London: Chatto & Windus.

94. Suzor, J. R. (1888). Exposé pratique du traitement de la rage par la méthode Pasteur: Historique et description de la rage, collection complète des communications de M. Pasteur, technique de sa méthode, resultats statistiques, etc. Paris: A. Maloine.

95. Weiss, R. (1924). La commémoration du centenaire de Pasteur par la Ville de Paris. Paris: Impr. nationale.

96. Dubos, R. (1950). Louis Pasteur: Free lance of science. Boston: Little, Brown and Company.

97. Ehrlich, P. and Norgenroth, J. (1899). Zur theorie der lysinwirkung. Berliner klin Wochenschr 1. (?).

98. Huxham, J. (1750). An essay on fevers: And their various kinds, as depending on different constitutions of the blood: with dissertations on slow nervous fevers; on putrid, pestilential, spotted fevers; on the small-pox; and on pleurisies and peripneumonies. London: S. Austen.

99. Jenner, E., & Parry, C. H. (1822). A letter to Charles Henry Parry: ... on the influence of artificial eruptions in certain diseases incidental to the human body, with an inquiry respecting the probable advantages to be derived from further experiments. London: Baldwin, Cradock, and Joy.

100. Jenner, E., & Drewitt, F. D. (1931). The note-book of Edward Jenner: In the possession of the Royal college of physicians of London. London: Oxford University Press, H. Milford.

101. Jones, W. H. S. (1909). Malaria and Greek history. Manchester: The University press.

102. Frankland, P. (1898). Pasteur. New York: The Macmillan Company.

103. Pfizer (Chas.) and Company, Inc., & Pasteur, L. (1958). New York: Pfizer.

104. The Pasteur fermentation centennial, 1857-1957: A scientific symposium on the occasion of the one hundredth anniversary of the publication of Louis Pasteur's Mémoire sur la fermentation appelée lactique. Hoppe-Seyler's Zeitschrift für physiologische Chemie. (1896). Strassburg: K.J. Trübner. (2 volumes)

105. Pasteur, L. (1848). Reserches sur le dimorphisme. Annales de Chimie et de Physique *3(23)*.

106. Pasteur, L. (1848). Reserches sur les relations qui peuvent exister entre la forme cristalline, la composition chimique et le sens de la polarisation rotatoire. Annales de Chimie et de Physique *3(24)*.

107. Pasteur, L. (1850). Recherches sur les proprietes specifiques des deux acides qui composent l'acide racemique. Annales de Chimie et de Physique *3(28)*.

108. Pasteur, L. (1851). Memoire dur les acides aspartique et malique.

109. Pasteur, L. (1853). Nouveaux faits relatifs a l'histoire de l'acide racemique (Lettre de M. Kestner a M. Biot). Comptes rendus des seances de l'Academie des Sciences *36*.

110. Pasteur, L. (1853). Recherches sur les alcaloides des quinquinas. Comptes rendus des seances de l'Academie des Sciences *37*.

111. Pasteur, L. (1853). Transformation des acides tartriques en acide racemique. Decouverte de l'acide tartrique inactif. Nouvelle methode de separation de l'acide racemique en acides tartriques droit et gauche. Comptes rendus des seances de l'Academie des Sciences 37.

112. Pasteur, L. (1854). Sur le dimorphisme dans les substances actives tetartoedrie. Annales de Chimie et de Physique *3(42)*.

113. Pasteur, L. (1856). Notice des travaux. Paris: Imprimerie de Mallet-Bachelier.

114. Pasteur, L. (1856). Etudes sur les modes d'accroissement des cristaux et sur les causes des variations de leurs formes secondaires. Annales de Chimie et de Physique 3(49).

115. Pasteur, L. (1853). Nouvelles recherches sur les relations que peuvent exister entre la forme cristalline, la composition chimique et le phenomene rotatoire moleculaire.

116. Pasteur, L. (1860). Recherches sur la dissymetrie moleculaire des produits organiques naturels. Lecons Professees a la Societe Chimique de Paris.

117. Pasteur, L. (1860). Recherches sur le mode de nutrition des mucedinees.

118. Pasteur, L. (1861). Notice des travaux. Annales de chimie et de physique 3(24).

119. Pasteur, L. (1860). Suite a une precedente communication relative aux generations dites spintanees.

120. Pasteur, L. (1861). Sur les corpuscules organisés qui existent dans l'atmosphère. Examen de la doctrine des générations spontanées.

121. Pasteur, L. (1864). Animalcules infusoires vivant sans gaz oxygene libre et determinant des fermentations. Paris: Imprimeur-Libraire Mallet-Bachelier.

122. Lettre adressee par M. Pasteur aux redacteurs des Annales de Chimie et de Physique. *(1861)*.

123. Pasteur, L. (1862). Memoire sur la fermentation acetique. Annales scientifiques de l'Ecole Normale superieure 1.

124. Pasteur, L. (1862). Nouveau procede industriel de fabrication du vinaigre. Paris: Imprimeur-Libraire Mallet-Bachelier.

125. Pasteur, L. (1862). Etudes sur les mycodermes. Role de ces plantes dans la fermentation acetique.

126. Pasteur, L. (1862). Notice de travaux. Paris: Imprimeur-Libraire Mallet-Bachelier.

127. Pasteur, L. (1863). Nouvel exemple de fermentation determinee par des animalcules infusoires pouvant vivre sans gaz oxygene libre, et en dehors de tout contact avec l'air de l'atmoshpère. Comptes rendus des seances de l'Academie de Sciences 56.

128. Pasteur, L. (1863). Examen du role attribue au gaz oxygene atmospherique dans la destruction des matieres animales et vegetales apres la mort. Comptes rendus des seances de l'Academie des Sciences 56.

129. Pasteur, L. (1863). Recherches sur la putrefactio. Comptes rendus des seances de l'Academie des Sciences 56.

130. Pasteur, L. (1863). Etudes sur les vins. Premiere partie: De l'influence de l'oxydene de l'air dans la vinification. Comptes rendus des seances de l'Academie des Sciences 57.

131. Pasteur, L. (1864). Etudes sur les vins. Deuxieme partie: Des alterations spontanees ou maladies des vins, particulierement dans le jura. Comptes rendus des seances de l'Academie des Sciences 58.

132. Pasteur, L. (1865). Procede pratique de conservation et d'amelioration des vins. Comptes rendus des seances de l'Academie des Sciences 60.

133. Pasteur, L. (1865). Note sur les depots qui se forment dans les vins. Comptes rendus des seances de l'Academie des Sciences 60.

134. Pasteur, L. (1865). Nouvelles observations au sujet de la conservation des vins. Comptes rendus des seances de l'Academie des Sciences 61.

135. Pasteur, L. (1865). Observations sur la maladie des vers a soie. Comptes rendus des seances de l'Academie des Sciences 61.

136. Pasteur, L. (1865). Sur la conservation des vins: Lettre adressee a M. Le Redacteur en chef du Moniteur Vinicole. Paris: Typographie de Henri Plon.

137. Pasteur, L. (1866). Nouvelles etudes sur la maladie des vers a soie. Comptes rendus des seances de l'Academie des Sciences 63.

138. Pasteur, L. (1866). Nouvelles etudes experimentales sur la maladie des vers a soie. Comptes rendus des seances de l'Academie des Sciences 63.

139. Pasteur, L. (1866). Observation verbales presentees apres la lecture de la note de M. A. Donne. Comptes rendus des seances de l'Academie des Sciences 63.

140. Quesneville, M. (1866). Conservation des vins: Lettre de M. Pasteur. Paris: Gauthier-Villars, Imprimeur-Libraire.

141. Pasteur, L. (1867). Nouvelle note sur la maladie des vers a soie. Epreuve.

142. Pasteur, L. and Dumas, M. (1868). Educations precoces de graines des races indigenes provenant de chambrees choisies. Comptes rendus des seances de l'Academie des Sciences 66.

143. Pasteur, L. (1868). Le budget de la science. Paris: Gauthier-Villars, Imprimeur-Libraire.

144. Pasteur, L. (1868). Rapport a son excellence m. le ministre de l'agriculture, du commerce et des travaux publics sur la mission confiee a M. Pasteur, en 1868. Relativement a la maladie des vers a soie. Paris: Imprimerie Imperiale.

145. Pasteur, L. (1869). Sériciculture: Note sur la sélection des cocons faite par le microscope pour la régénération des races indigènes de vers à soie. Comptes rendus des séances de l'Académie des Sciences 69.

146. Pasteur, L. (1869). De la pratique du chauffage pour la conservation et l'amélioration des vins. Comptes rendus des séances de l'Académie des Sciences 69.

147. Pasteur, L. (1869). Note relative aux communications de M. de Vergnette-Lamotte et de M. P. Thenard adressées à l'Académie dans les séances des 20 septembre et 4 octobre. Comptes rendus des séances de l'Académie des Sciences 69.

148. Pasteur, L. (1870). Rapport: Adressé à l'Académie ser les résultats des éducations pratiques de ver à soie, effectuées au moyen de graines préparées par les procédés de sélection. Comptes rendus des séances de l'Académie des Sciences 71.

149. Pourquoi la France n'a pas trouvé d'hommes supérieurs au moment du péril. Rome 1871

150. Pasteur, L. (1871). Quelques réflexions sur la science en France. Paris: Gauthier-Villars, Imprimeur-Libraire.

151. Perraud, J.J. (1876). Discours de M. Pasteur. Paris: Typographie de Firmin Didot.

152. Pasteur, L. and Joubert. (1877). Charbon et speticémie. Comptes rendus des séances de l'Académie des Sciences 85. (2 copies)

153. Pasteur, L. (1878). La théorie des germes et ses applications a la médecine et la chirurgie. Paris.

154. Pasteur, L. (1880). Sur l'étiologie du charbon. Comptes rendus des sèances de l'Académie des Sciences 91.

155. Pasteur, L. (1881). Sur la longue durée de la vie des germes charbonneux et sur leur conservation dans les terres cultivées. Comptes rendus des sèances de l'Académie des Sciences 92.

156. Pasteur, L. (1881). De l'atténuation des virus et de leur retour à la virulence. Comptes rendus des sèances de l'Académie des Sciences 92.

157. Pasteur, L. (1881). Sur la vaccination charbonneuse. Paris: Gauthier-Villars, Imprimeur-Libraire.

158. Discours de Professeur Pasteur. 1881

159. (1882). Disours prononcé dans la séance publique tenue par l'Académie Française pour la réception de M. Pasteur. Paris: Typographie de Firmin-Didot.

160. Pasteur, L. (1882). Sur le rouget, ou mal rouge des procs. Comptes rendus des séances de l'Académie des Sciences 95.

161. Pasteur, L. (1883). De l'atténuation des virus. Quartrième congrés international d'hygiène et de démographie.

162. Pasteur, L. (1883). La vaccination charbonneuse. Paris: Germer Bailliere.

163. Pasteur, L. (1883). Les doctrines dites microbiennes et la vaccination charbonneuse. Extrait du Bulletin de l'Académie de Médecine.

164. Pasteur, L. and Thuillier (1883). La vaccination du rouget des porcs à l'aide du virus mortel atténué de cette maladie. Comptes rendus des séances de l'Académie des Sciences 97.

165. Pasteur, L. (1884). Sur la rage. Comptes rendus des séances de l'Académie des Sciences 98.

166. Pasteur, L. (1884). Nouvelle communication sur la rage. Comptes rendus des séances de l'Académie des Sciences 98.

167. Bertrand, J. (1885). Réponse de M. Pasteur directeur de l'Académie Française.

168. Pasteur, L. (1886). Résultats de l'application de la méthode pour prévenir la rage. Paris: Gauthier-Villars, Imprimeur-Libraire.

169. Pasteur, L. (1886). Note complémentaire sur les résultats de l'application de la méthode de prophylaxie de la rage. Paris: Gauthier-Villars, Imprimeur-Libraire.

170. Pasteur, L. (1886). Nouvelle communication sur la rage. Paris: Gauthier-Villars, Imprimeur-Libraire.

171. Pasteur, L. (1889). Inauguration de la statue de J. B. Dumas.

172. Pasteur, L. (1849). Reserches sur les proprietes specifiques des deux acides qui composent l'acide racemique. Comptes renduus des seances de l'Academie des Sciences 29.

173. Pasteur, L. (1850). Nouvelles recherches sur les relations qui peuvent exister, entre la forme cristalline, la composition chimique, et le pouvior rotatoire moleculaire. Comptes rendus des seances de l'Academie des Sciences 31.

174. Pasteur, L. (1851). Relatif aux acides aspartique et malique. Comptes rendus des seances de l'Academie des Sciences 33.

175. Pasteur, L. (1853). Nouvelles recherches sur les relations qui peuvent exister entre la forme cristalline, la composition chimique et le phenomene rotatoire moleculaire. Comptes rendus des seances de l'Academie des Sciences 36.

176. Extrait du rapport sur le concours pour le prix de physiologie experimentale pour l'annee (1859). Comptes rendus des seances de l'Academie des Sciences 50.

177. Discours prononces sur la tomee de M. Isidore Geoffroy Saint-Hilaire. (1861). Paris: Imprimerie de L. Martinet.

178. Rapport sur le prix Jecker, annee (1861). Comptes rendus des seances de l'Academie des Sciences 53.

179. Rapport sur les experiences relatives a la generation spontanee. (1865). Comptes rendus des seances de l'Academie des Sciences 60.

180. Soret, J.L. (1867). Recherches sur la densite de l'ozone. Geneve: Imprimerie Ramboz et Schuchardt.

181. Pasteur, L. (1873). Note sur les travaux. Paris: Imprimerie de Gauthier-Villars.

182. Pasteur, L. (1874). Compte-rendu de la distribution des prix. Arbois.

183. Lévéque, Ch. (1874). Séance publique annuelle. Paris: Typographie de Firmin Didot Frères.

184. Pasteur, L. (1880). D'étuves publiques pour la désinfection des objets de literie et des linges qui ont été en contact avec des personnes atteintes de maladies infecteuses ou contagieuses. Paris: Typographie Charles de Mourgues Frères.

185. (1888). Inauguration de l'Institut Pasteur. Seaux: Charaire et Fils.

186. 5 page handwritten letter

187. Baillet, C.C. (1872). Notice sur les titres et travaux scientifiques. Corbell: Typographie de Crété Fils.

188. Report of a committee appointed by the local government board to inquire into M. Pasteur's treatment of hydrophobia. London: Harrison and Sons.

189. Letter requesting permission to deliver a paper before the Academie des Sciences. 1857

190. 4 page letter. 1859

191. Cover letter for list of expenses for Pasteur's lab, which the government has undertaken to pay. 1859

192. Pasteur's process for making acetic acid- a component of vinegar. 1861

193. Requests financial aid for research work, which Pasteur had been paying for out of his own pocket until now. 1864

194. Letter to M. Lanqentin, President of the Wine Trade Committee, giving details of Pasteur's researches on wine and asking for support. 1865

195. Eloquent plea for government funding of the building of a new bio-chemistry lab at the Ecole normale, which will be placed under Pasteur's direction.

196. Bouley, H. (1881). Sur les travaux de M. Pasteur. Paris: Typographie de V. Renou, Maulde, et Cock.

197. Requests the minister's approval of a new position for René Guillemot, President of the Civil Tribunal of Rion.

198. 2 page letter concerning rabies. 1887

199. 43 pages concerning Pasteur's work on rabies. 1888

200. (1895). *Ludwig Pasteur.*

201. Appréciations de M. le professor Koch, de Berlin, sur les travaux de M. Pasteur.

202. Boutroux, L. (1881). Sur l'habitat et la conservation des levûres spontanées. Caen: Imprimerie de F. le Blanc-Hardel.

203. Chamberland, Ch. (1879). Thèses presentées a la faculté de sciences de Paris pour le grade de docteur ès sciences physiques. Paris: Gauthier-Villars, Imprimeur-Libraire.

204. Chamberland, Ch. (1879). Résistance des germes de certains organismes à la température de 100 degrés; conditions de leur développement.

205. Chamberland, Ch. (1882). Role de microbes dans la production des maladies. Paris: Gauthier-Villars, Imprimeur-Libraire.

206. Recherches historiques sur l'étiologie et la contagion des affections charbonneuses. Sociéte de Médecine Vétérinaire.

207. Chauveu, A. (1883). De la préparation et du mode d'emploi des cultures atténuées par le chauffage, pour servir aux inoculations préventives contre le charbon. Comptes rendus des séances de l'Académie des Sciences 97.

208. Chauveau, J.B. (1877). Thèse pour le doctorat en médecine: Contribution a l'étude de la vaccine originelle. Paris: Libraire Germer Baillière et Cie.

209. Chauveau, A. (1880). Du rendorcement de l'immunité des moutons algériens, à l'égard du sang de rate, par les inoculaitons préventives. Influences de l'inoculation

de la mère sur la réceptivité du fœtus. Comptes rendus des séances de l'Académie des Sciences 91.

210. Chauveau, A. (1880). Sur la résistance des animaux de l'espèce bovine au sang de rate et sur la préservation de ces animaux par les inoculations préventives. Comptes rendus des séances de l'Académie des Sciences 91.

211. Chauveau, A. (1881). De l'atténuation des effets des inoculations virulentes par l'emloi de très petites quantités de virus. Comptes rendus des séances de l'Académie des Sciences 92.

212. Chauveau, A. (1884). De la préparation en grandes masses des cultures atténuées par le chauffage rapide pour l'inoculation préventive du sang de rate. Comptes rendus des séances de l'Académie des Sciences 98.

213. Joly, N. (1862). Examen critique du mémoire de M. Pasteur relatif aux générations spontanées. Moniteur scientifique. Quesneville.

214. Rossignol, H. (1881). Rapport sur les expériences de pouilly-le-fort. Melun: Imprimerie Typographie E. Drosne.

215. Roux, E. (1883). Nouvelles acquisitions sur la rage. Paris: A. Parent, Imprimeur de la Faculté de Médecine.

216. Roux, E. Croonian Lecture: Les incoulations préventives.

217. Bernard, Claude (1813-1878). A collection of 10 fine quality photographic enlargements reproducing all of the best original photographs of Claude Bernard, the statures honoring him in France, and a portrait painting. Eight of these ten black-and-white prints are skillfully mounted on white matt board (16 ¾ x 13 ¾ inches).

218. Pasteur. Portrait etching by Louis Orr after the painting by Albert Edelfelt (1854-1905). 55 x 44cm in plate, with margins extending to 63 x 48cm.

219. Collection of picture postcards documenting his life, portraiture.

220. Hand-colored aquatint. Reduced version of etching by Albert Edelfelt.

221. Portrait engraving by Champollion.

222. Autographed letter signed, framed with photograph of Pasteur and hand-colored photo of bas-relief illustrating Pasteur's experiments with rabies.

223. Beddoes, T. (1799). Essay on the causes, early signs, and prevention of pulmonary consumption for the use of parents and preceptors. London: Longman and Rees.

224. Davaine, C.-J. (1860). Traité des entozoaires et des maladies vermineuses de l'homme et des animaux domestiques. Paris: J.B. Baillière et fils.

225. Dubos, R. J. (1950). Louis Pasteur, free lance of science. Boston: Little, Brown.

226. Ehrlich, P., Hata, S., Newbold, A., & Felkin, R. W. (1911). The experimental chemotherapy of spirilloses: (syphilis, relapsing fever, spirillosis of fowls, framboesia. London: Rebman.

227. Naegeli, O. (1913). Leukaemie und pseudoleukaemie. Leipzig: Alfred Hölder.

228. Fleming, A. (1946). Penicillin, its practical application. Philadelphia: Blakiston.

229. Hecker, J. F. C., & Babington, B. G. (1846). The epidemics of the middle ages. London: G. Woodfall and Son.

230. Ashburn, P. M. (1929). A History of the Medical Department of the United States Army. Boston and New York: Houghton Mifflin Company.

231. Bardsley, J. L. (1830). Hospital facts and observations: Illustrative of the efficacy of the new remedies, strychnia, brucia, acetate of morphia, veratria, iodine, &c. in several morbid conditions of the system: with a comparative view of the treatment of chorea, and some cases of diabetes: a report on the efficacy of sulphureous fumigations in diseases of the skin, chronic rheumatism, &c. London: Burgess and Hill.

232. Bayle, G. L., & Stanton A. Friedberg, M.D. Rare Book Collection of Rush University Medical Center at the University of Chicago. (1810). Recherches sur la phthisie pulmonaire: Ouvrage lu à la société de la Faculté de médecine de Paris, dans diverses séances, en 1809 et 1810. Paris: Gabon.

233. Bazin, E. (1861). Leçons théoriques et cliniques sur la scrofule: Considérée en elle-même et dans ses rapports avec la syphilis, la dartre et l'arthritis. Paris: Delahaye.

234. Beddoes, T. (1803). Observations on the medical and domestic management of the consumptive: On the powers of digitalis purpurea; and on the cure of schrophula. Troy, N.Y.: Printed by O. Penniman and Co.; sold by them at the Troy bookstore, and by Richards and Bliss, Utica.

235. Bernard, C. (1857). Leçons sur les effets des substances toxiques et médicamenteuses. Paris: Baillière.

236. Carpenter, W. B. & Smith, F. G. (1856). The microscope and its revelations. Philadelphia: Blanchard and Lea.

237. Cheyne, W. W. S. (1886). Recent essays by various authors on bacteria in relation to disease: Selected and edited by *W.W. Cheyne*. London.

238. Coxe, J. R. & Humphreys, J. (1802). Practical observations on vaccination: Or inoculation for the cow-pock. Philadelphia: Printed and sold by James Humphreys.

239. Currie, J., Humphreys, J., & Benjamin & Thomas Kite (Firm). (1808). Medical reports, on the effects of water, cold and warm, as a remedy in fever and other diseases: Whether applied to the surface of the body, or used internally. Philadelphia: Printed for James Humphreys, and for Benjamin and Thomas Kite.

240. Ehrlich, P., & Lazarus, A. (1898). Die Anaemie. Wien: A. Hölder.

241. Ehrlich, P., Lazarus, A. and Pinkus, F. (1901). Leukaemie, pseudoleikaemie, haemeglobinaemie. Wien: A. Hölder.

242. In Ehrlich, P., In Mosse, M., In Krause, R., In Rosin, H., & In Weigert, K. (1903). Encyklopädie der mikrospischen Technik: Mit besonderer Berücksichtigung der Färbelehr. Berlin [Urban & Schwarzenberg].

243. Ehrlich, P. (1906). Arbeiten aus dem königlichen institut für experimentelle therapie zu Frankfurt A.M. Jena: Verlag von Gustav Fischer.

244. Ehrlich, P. (1911). Abhandlungen über Salvarsan. München: Lehmann. (4 volumes)

245. Apolant, H. (1914). Paul Ehrlich, eine Darstellung seines wissenschaftlichen Wirkens. Jena: Fischer.

246. Fleming, A., & H.K. Lewis and Company. (1929). On the antibacterial action of cultures of a penicillium, with special reference to their use in the isolation of B. influenzae. London: H.K. Lewis.

247. Fontana, F. (1767). Ricerche fisiche sopra il veleno della vipera. In Lucca: Nella stamperìa di Jacopo Giusti.

248. Hennen, J., & Hennen, J. (1830). Sketches of the medical topography of the Mediterranean: Comprising an account of Gibraltar, the Ionian Islands, and Malta. London: Thomas and George Underwood.

249. Holmes, O. W., National Center for Homoeopathy (U.S.), American Foundation for Homoeopathy, & Stanton A. Friedberg, M.D. Rare Book Collection of Rush University Medical Center at the University of Chicago. (1861). Currents and counter-currents in medical science: With other addresses and essays. Boston: Ticknor and Fields.

250. Duclaux, E. (1886). Le microbe et la maladie. Paris: Masson.

251. Ehrlich, P. (1884). Aus der klinik des wirkl. geh. ober-med-rath Professor Dr. v Frerichs. Ueber die sulfodiazobenzol-reaction.

252. Ehrlich, P. (1885). Antikritische bemerkungen über drüsenfunctionen.

253. Ehrlich, P. (1885). Das Sauerstoff-Bedürfniss des Organismus: Eine farbenanalytische Studie. Berlin: Hirschwald.

254. Ehrlich, P. and Laquer, B. (1885). Ueber continuirliche thallinzuführung und deren wirkung beim abdominaltyphus.

255. Ehrlich, P. (1886). Aus der klinik des herrn geheimrath Professor Dr. Gerhardt. Experimentelles und klinisches über thallin. Deutschen Medicinischen Wochenschrift 48(50).

256. Ehrlich, P. (1886). Beiträge zur theorie der bacillenfärbung. Berlin: Verlag von August Hirschwald.

257. Ehrlich, P. (1890). Studien in der cocainreihe. Leipzig: Verlag von Georg Thieme.

258. Ehrlich, P. (1891). Farbenanalytische Untersuchungen zur Histologie und Klinik des Blutes: Gesammelte Mittheilungen. Berlin: August Hirschwald.

259. Ehrlich, P. (1891). Experimentelle untersuchungen über immunität. Leipzig: Verlag von Georg Thieme.

260. Ehrlich, P. (1891). Experimentelle untersuchungen über immunität. Deutschen Medicinischen Wochenschrift 44.

261. Guttmann, P. & Ehrlich, P. (1891). Ueber die wirkung des methylenblau bei malaria. Sonderabdruck aus Berliner klin. Wochenschrift 39.

262. Ehrlich, P. (1893). Constitution, Vertheilung und Wirkung chemischer Koerper: Aeltere und neuere arbeiten. Leipzig: G. Thieme.

263. Ehrlich, P. (1897). Die wertbemessung des diphtherieheilserums und deren theoretische grundlagen. Jena: Verlag von Gustav Fischer.

264. Ehrlich, P. (1898). Ueber die beziehungen von chemischer constitution, vertheilung und pharmakologischer wirkung.

265. Ehrlich, P. (1898). Ueber die constitution des diphtheriegiftes. Leipzig: Verlag von Georg Thieme.

266. Ehrlich, P. (1899). Mode d'action et mécanisme de production des antitoxines. Paris: Imprimerie de la Semaine Médicale.

267. Ehrlich, P. (1899). Observations upon the constitution of the diphtheria toxin. London: John Bale, Sons & Danielsson, Ltd.

268. Ehrlich, P. and Morgenroth, J. (1899). Ueber haemolysine. Diese Wochenschrift 1.

269. Ehrlich, P. (1900). Toxines et antitoxines. Paris: XIII Congres International de Médecine.

270. Ehrlich, P., Lazarus, A., & Myers, W. (1900). Histology of the blood: Normal and pathological. Cambridge [Eng.: University Press.

271. Ehrlich, P. (1900). On immunity with special reference to cell life. London.

272. Ehrlich, P. and Morgenroth, J. (1901). Ueber Hämolysine. Sonderabdruck aus der Berliner klin. Wochenschr. 10.

273. Ehrlich, P. and Morgenroth, J. (1901). Ueber Hämolysine. Sonderabdruck aus der Berliner klin. Wochenschr. 21 and 22.

274. Ehrlich, P. (1901). Schlussbetrachtungen. Wien: Alfred Hölder.

275. Ehrlich, P. (1901). Die schutzstoffe des blutes. Leipzig: Verlag von F.C.W. Vogel.

276. Ehrlich, P. and Sachs, H. (1902). Ueber die vielheit der complemente des serums. Sonderabdruck aus der Berliner klinischen Wochenschrift 14 and 15.

277. Ehrlich, P. and Sachs, H. (1902). Ueber den mechanismus der amboceptorenwirkung. Sonderabdruck aus der Berliner klin. Wochenschr. 21.

278. Ehrlich, P. and Marshall, H.T. (1902). Ueber die complementophilen gruppen der amboceptoren. Sonderabdruck aus der Berliner klin. Wochenschr. 25.

279. Ehrlich, P. (1903). Mechanismus der ambozeptorwirkung und seine teleologische bedeutung. Jena: Verlag von Gustav Fischer.

280. Ehrlich, P. (1903). Ueber die giftcomponenten des diphtheria-toxins. Sonderabdruck aus der Berliner klinischen Wochenschrift 35-37.

281. Ehrlich, P. (1903). Toxin und antitoxin. Sonderabdruck aus der Berliner klinischen Wochenschrift 33 and 34.

282. Ehrlich, P. (1904). Farbentherapeutische versuche bei trypanosomenerkrankung. Sonderabdruck aus der Berliner klinischen Wochenschrift 13 and 14.

283. Ehrlich, P. (1904). Gesammelte Arbeiten zur Immunitätsforschung. Berlin: Hirschwald.

284. Ehrlich, P. and Herter, C.A. (1904). Physiologische chemie. Strassburg: Verlag von Karl J. Trübner.

Reynolds-Finley Historical Library, University of Alabama in Birmingham

Descriptions provided by Reynolds-Finley Historical Library.

1. *Pour le vieillir par M. L. Pasteur…* deuxiéme edition revue et augmentée avec 32 planches imprimées en couleur et 25 gravures dans le texte. Paris, Librairie F. Savy, 1873. [Ms. writing in ink.] Ff. 142 + additional blank pages. Ms. prepared in a legible hand, apparently for the printer. Four of the plates are original and drawn in color.

2. Holograph letter to M. Bousson mentioning Jean Baptiste Biot, French physicist, who had just died. On paper with letterhead of Ecole Normale Supérieure, Université de France. Feb. 9, 1862.

3. Letter written in ink by Louis Pasteur to "Mon cher confrère" about the creation of a chair of organic chemistry for Berthelot, and Bernard and the lack of a chair of experimental physiology. On paper with letterhead of Ecole Normale Supérieure, Université de France. Paris, Dec. 23, 1863.

4. Letters on silkworm disease, written to M. Jeanjean. Dated Paris and Alais, April 9, 1866-June 7, 1889. 20 holograph letters.

5. Eight letters written by Mme. Pasteur, seven of which are signed by Pasteur. Dated from 1868/69 when he was prevented from writing by his paralytic stroke.

6. Two visiting cards with autograph notes.

7. Two telegrams from Louis Pasteur.

8. One letter of Lachadenede's, July 21, 1866.

9. One official letter from the Legion of Honor, July 11, 1882.

10. Letter of April 1, 1867 is from M. Delesse to Pasteur. Pasteur's to Jeanjean is on verso.

11. Letter to Jules Léonard Raulin from Lyon written in ink by Louis Pasteur, on his future work, and his refusal of Signor Chiozza's offer to work in Pisa. Dated Lyons, Feb. 13, 1871.

12. Holograph letter signed L. Pasteur, to M. Marchand of Dijon, on his dog's rabies. Dated Paris, Aug. 12, 1881. [Accompanying addressed envelope with canceled postage stamp.]

13. Seventeen Letters written in ink by Louis Pasteur to "mon cher Thuillier" on anthrax, chicken cholera, rouget, vaccination of animals. Dated Paris and Arbois, April 15, 1882-Aug. 6, 1883.

14. Letter written in ink by L. Pasteur to "cher professeur" on the satisfactory results of anthrax vaccination and the experiment at Pouilly le Fort. Dated Paris, July 20, 1888. [On green paper with initials L. P.]

15. Holograph note on rabies: "De toutes les maladies virulentes, la rage est la plus facile à prévenir." Signed L. Pasteur. Institut Pasteur, no date.

16. [Black and white] Portraits of Louis Pasteur and unidentified friend, undated. 2 photos. 7 ½ X 10 ½ cm., 7 X 5 cm. [2 reproductions also included] Autograph note on the back of the larger photograph. Unpublished photos.

17. [Black and white] Portrait of Louis Pasteur dictating to Mme. Pasteur, photo undated. 1 photo. 12 ½ X 18 cm.

18. Hubert, Eugène, b. 1839. *Quelques pages de déontologie médicale.* Lierre: Typ. de Joseph van In et cie, 1892. [Reynolds Library copy has author's presentation inscription to Pasteur on the endpaper: "À Pasteur / hommage [illegible] de Eugène Hubert".]

Huntington Library in San Mateo, California
Descriptions provided by Huntington Library.

1. Pasteur, Louis. 1 Oct 1888

2. Sur les Fermentations [1860]

3. Manuscript draft of first report to French Academy of Sciences on use of rabies vaccine on humans

4. Pasteur notes

5. Pasteur

6. Letter proposing use of anthrax virus to control rabbit population in Australia. 1 Oct. 1988

7. Fermentation

8. Manuscript draft of first report to French Academy of Sciences on use of rabies vaccine in humans

9. Notes pour Leçon sur la cellulose. 1854 Avril

10. Note sur l'inversion du sucre de cannes dans la fermentation alcoulique

11. Passage d'un Compte Rendu de M. Foucault. 11 Jullet 1860

12. Sur les Corpuscules Organisés qui Existent dans l'Atmosphère 1861

13. Pasteur, Louis a S.E. le Minotre d'Etat. 13 Avril 1861

14. Sur les fermentations [1861?]

15. Lettre de M. Pasteur …. a M. Quesneville. 1866

16. La Vie c'est la Germe avec son Devenir et le Germe c'est la vie [1870?]

17. Pasteur- Premiere Conclusion du Cangus Sericole International. 1870

18. Bulletin de l'Union Médicale. Jeudi 18 Fevrier 1875

19. La Theorie des Germes... 30 Avril 1878

20. Réponse a M. Berthelot… 30 decembre 1878

21. Vies sur les Epidemes Resultant de ma Lectare dumardi. 26 Octobre [1880]

22. Rédaction Paur Une Réponse… a M. Chauveau. 31 Octobre [1880]

23. Sure la durée de la préservation du choléra des poules. Avril 1881

24. Pasteur, Louis. 22 Mai 1881

25. Sur las Vaccination Charbonneuse. 13 Juni 1881

26. International Medical Congress. Discours de Professor Pasteur. 8 about 1881

27. [sur l'attenuation des virus] 11 novembre 1881

28. sur le rouget, ou mal rouge des pores. 4 decembre 1882

29. de l'influence des milieux de culture... 17 octobre 1884

30. sur la destruction des lapins en Australie... 5 janvier 1888

31. a propos de la fete du 27 decembre 1892… 1893

32. Photographies Originales des Premiers Personnes Vaccines contra la rage. 1885

33. Photographies Originales de Pasteur. 1868, 1881, 1889

34. "Projet de Toast du Banquet du 17" Avril 1884

35. Pasteur, Louis. 22 mars [1885]

36. Pasteur, Louis. Janv 1887

37. Pasteur, Louis. 20 Sept (?).

38. Etude sur les maladies transmissibles. 2 mai 1877

39. sur la rage [1886]

40. Pasteur, Louis. 5 mars 1888

41. "Discours pronone aux fetes du tricentenaire de l'Universite d'Edinbourg" [1884]

42. Pasteur, Louis. 6 Juli 1886

43. Pasteur, Louis. Telegramme, 4 novembre 1885

44. Pasteur, Louis. 26 feurier 1885

45. Notes pour servir discours de reception a l'Academie Francaise en 1882

46. Pasteur, Louis. 1885

47. de L'ougne de ferments organises. 7 juin 1876

48. Pasteur, Louis. 6 novembre 1884

49. Bases d'un rappoit a faire avant la rentre de 1859-60. 30 juin 1859

50. Pasteur, Louis. 2 mars 1887

51. a-b "Discours de reception a l'Academie Francaise" 27 Avril 1882

52. Pasteur, Louis. 18 Novembre 1857

53. sur l'Ecole Normale. 1860

54. Advertisement. 12 avril 1864.

55. Pasteur, Louis. 9 dec 1882

56. Pasteur, Louis. 23 juin 1888

57. Pasteur, Louis. 31 August 1886

58. "Reponse au discours de M. J. Bertraurd…" [10 dec 1895]

59. deux notes

60. re: M. Chauveau et la rage

61. extrait de l'elage de Hauy par Cuvier

62. "Note pour Fernin et Eugene" 23 juillet 1889

63. note

64. note written on envelope

65. note

66. note

67. note

68. note. 26 July 1884

69. Pasteur, Louis. 8 janvier 1888

70. Pasteur, Louis

71. Pasteur, Louis. 3 August 1888

72. Pasteur, Louis. 24 Avril

73. Pasteur, Louis. 19 Nov 1884

74. Memoire sur la cause et les effets de la fermentation alcoolique et acceteuse par M. Turpin. 1860?

75. Cells. 1873

76. Dinér chez la princesse Mathilde

77. a-b epreuves corriges d'un texte institute "Les Laboratories" with "Le Budge de la Science" 1868

78. Sur la nage et vivesection

79. Sur les vins de Corse. 7 August 1876

80. Pasteur, Louis. 31 July 1883

81. "Notes académiques"

82. Sur Lavoisier. 1774

83. Extract from Berzelius. 1841

84. "Resultats de Quelques de mes essais..." 1856

85. Comptes rendus. 1864

86. Comptes rendu. 1863

87. Chemical notes

88. "Messieurs... Nous avons"

89. "Personnes traites et en traitment..." 18 juillet 1886

90. Re: M. Coudé agé de 25 ans. 1885

91. Note sur l'Etat Déplorable de la Sériculture en France. 1877

92. Note

93. Pasteur, Louis. 16 Jan 1888

94. Pasteur, Louis. 5 January 1888

95. Sur la cristallisation. 1788

96. "Stahl – Fermentation" and notes on chemistry

97. prefecture de Police – Cons. d'Hygiene. 188?

98. Research notes

99. "Vins, raisins". 10 April 1872

100. 6 photos

101. 3 cards. 16 January 1885

102. Descriptions (past 20 folders)

103. Descriptions

104. Notes; la Societe Holland ause des Sciences. 1869

105. Notes; Addresses a M. le Ministere de l'Instruction Publique. 6 Mai 1858

106. Pasteur, Louis. 24 Janvier 1876

107. Pasteur, Louis. 11 Juin 1888

108. Pasteur, Louis. 4 February 1879

109. Pasteur, Louis. 26 Avril 1881

110. Pasteur, Louis. 6 Janvier 1881

111. Pasteur, Louis. 27 August 1880

112. Pasteur, Louis. 30 Mai 1880

113. Pasteur, Louis. 27 Mai 1880

114. Pasteur, Louis (draft "mon cheri ami")

115. Pasteur, Louis (draft of letter to M. Desseilligny)

116. Pasteur, Louis (fragment to Ministre de l'Instruction Publique)

117. Pasteur, Louis. 2 March 1868

118. Pasteur, Louis with C. Octavus Budd. 29 Oct 1863

119. Pasteur, Louis (draft of letter to Ministre de l'Instruction Publique)

120. Pasteur, Louis (draft of letter to Ministre de l'Instruction Publique)

121. Pasteur, Louis. 26 August 1865

122. Pasteur, Louis with C. Octavus Budd. 1865

123. Pasteur, Louis. 9 Dec 1866

124. Pasteur, Louis. 16 July 1867

125. Pasteur, Louis. 28 Sept 1869

126. Pasteur, Louis with the Compte de Saint Yricq 1862

127. Pasteur, Louis. 14 Nov 1855

128. Pasteur, Louis. 15 Nov 1855

129. Pasteur, Louis. 1856

130. Pasteur, Louis. 15 Nov 1855

131. Durvy, V. with M. D. Nisard. 1864-65

132. Pasteur, Louis. 3 Juin 1856

133. Maire de Lille a Doyen. 7 Juin 1856

134. Pasteur, Louis

135. Pasteur, Louis

136. Pasteur, Louis 20 Sept 1859

137. Pasteur, Louis 13 Dec 1859

138. Pasteur, Louis 19 Feb 1862

139. Pasteur, Louis 31 Dec 1856

140. Pasteur, Louis 3 Oct 1856

141. Pasteur, Louis. 1856

142. Note, Date?

143. Pasteur, Louis 23 Juillet 1867

144. Note "mon cher directeur"

145. Notes. 1863

146. Notes

147. Carte de visite de William P. Blake. Sept 1869

148. Memo a M. Prodhomme

149. Note

150. Pasteur, Louis 29 Sept 1888

151. Pasteur, Louis 7 Mai 1888

152. Pasteur, Louis (draft letter)

153. Pasteur, Louis 19 Mars 1879

154. a-b Pasteur collection information and provenance

155. a-d Pasteur Autographs

156. Sur la fermentation de la brere

157. Calmette's note to Pasteur, with responses in margin by Pasteur 1874

158. Sur la bere 18 Avril 1874

Harry Ransom Center, University of Texas.
Descriptions provided by Harry Ransom Center include the following.

1. Four autographed manuscripts of the first published study of Pasteur's life and work by René Vallery-Radot.

2. Manuscripts with corrections/additions by Pasteur.

3. Books with annotations by Pasteur.

4. Books inscribed to Pasteur.

5. Books by and about Pasteur.

6. Fifty mounted photographs and prints.

7. A pen-and-ink portrait of Pasteur by Dr. Emile Roux, signed by both.

www.ingramcontent.com/pod-product-compliance
Lightning Source LLC
Chambersburg PA
CBHW051410200326
41520CB00023B/7181